# VALUES OF PHYSICAL ACTIVITY

VALUES OF

# George J. Holland

*California State University, Northridge,
Executive Director, San Fernando
Valley Health Consortium*

# Elwood Craig Davis

*California State University, Northridge
Emeritus Professor, University of
Southern California*

# Foreword by R. K. Burke

*University of Southern California*

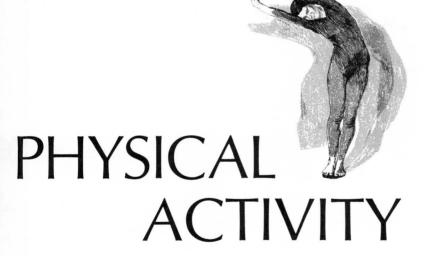

# PHYSICAL ACTIVITY

**Third Edition**

Wm. C. Brown Company Publishers
Dubuque, Iowa

Photographs by Dr. George Q. Rich III, Exercise Physiology
  Laboratory
Drawings by Saul Bernstein, Two Dimension Art Department,
  California State University, Northridge.

PHYSICAL EDUCATION

Consulting Editor
  *Aileene Lockhart*
  *Texas Woman's University*

HEALTH

Consulting Editor
  *Robert Kaplan*
  *The Ohio State University*

PARKS AND RECREATION

Consulting Editor
  *David Gray*
  *California State University, Long Beach*

Copyright © 1961 by Elwood Craig Davis and Gene A. Logan

Copyright © 1965, 1975 by Wm. C. Brown Company Publishers

Library of Congress Catalog Card Number: 74–12787

ISBN 0–697–07128–6

Printed in the United States of America

## TO

*All those who would
better understand and seek the many
values of physical activity*

# Contents

# Foreword

SOME YEARS ago, I shared-the-ride to my college teaching job each morning with a newly-appointed sociologist. He was curious about the nature of my duties as a professor of physical education, and over a period of time he quizzed me extensively as we drove along. In a skeptical but open-minded way, he asked me why I thought physical education activity courses should be offered in a liberal arts curriculum. Since he was a research specialist, I based my arguments almost exclusively on facts from exercise physiology, emphasizing the contributions of exercise to physical health and fitness. Then, one morning as I slid out of the car in front of the Physical Education Building, he hit me with a punchline: "You should get a quarter-mile-long treadmill—one that could be programmed automatically for daily increments of speed and duration. Group the students in homogeneous classes according to present level of fitness. Then put them on the treadmill, about a hundred at a time. Two staff members could handle it—one exercise physiologist to classify students and program the treadmill, and one technician to maintain machinery, monitor attendance, and certify final grades. The rest of the physical education faculty could be terminated, and . . . ." It was 7:59 A.M., and I lost the last part of his sentence as I dashed to my eight o'clock. Shortly afterwards, he moved, and I never had an opportunity to try to explain to him what physical education is really like.

But no matter. I know he was putting me on. As a competent sociologist, he had detected the insufficiency and narrowness of my interpretation of physical education.

Among those of us who are collegiate specialists and textbook writers, it is a common failing to become too narrowly preoccupied with the technical aspects of our subject matter. In self-defense, we could point out that the role of theoretical scholar or applied scientist is an essential one. In these closing years of the 20th Century, practicing professionals cannot compete successfully without a sophisticated knowledge of exercise physiology, kinesiology, biomechanics, and applied psychology. We live in an age of technology, and if we specialize in promoting excellence of human performance we cannot neglect the mechanistic aspects of human functioning.

But it is all too easy to become captured by the megatechnics of our time. As we discover cybernetic elements in human performance, it is all too easy to act as if humans *are* machines, forgetting that they are also emotional, creative, independent seekers of values and meaning. It is all too easy to write textbooks in which the factual or scientific subject matter is sterilized by the neglect of a crucial ingredient—*humanity*.

Happily, the book in hand, by George J. Holland and Elwood Craig Davis, is not a case in point. Its science, although authentic, is presented within a humanic context. Its philosophy is not didactic or doctrinal, but instead suggests processes and information for the reader to use in his or her own way. Science and philosophy are integrated so that objective information has guidelines for establishing values and deciding how to strive to achieve them. This makes this book unique in its field.

R. K. BURKE

# Preface

THE LIFE-style of college students is changing rapidly in the 1970s. Many young adults have seriously undertaken the task of building a new hierarchy of values and a new set of purposes for life and living. In the course of such a task, one philosophizes, that is, he or she uses the philosophic process. The student intellectually utilizes philosophic ingredients in considering and applying dependable evidence, such as scientifically-determined facts to such facets as his life-style, his possible vocational preferences, his relationships with others and his environment, and the level of physical-mental well-being he wishes to gain and to maintain.

College students are increasingly aware of an attempt to unify knowledge, both in the natural and social sciences and philosophy. This book represents an amalgamation, a synthesis of scientific inquiry and the philosophic quest. It is the planned intention of the authors to provide, in this book, a personal, rational basis for the evolvement of one important element of living. Biochemists, medical researchists, physiologists, sports medicine technicians, kinesiologists, motor psychologists, and researchers in physical education are uncovering, at a growing rate, scientific findings related to the effects of muscular activity upon the human male and female organism. This growing body of scientifically determined information must be adequately synthesized so that each individual can philosophically determine whether participation in the dance, exercise, or sports shall play an integral and desired part of his life-style today and tomorrow.

Part One of the book provides a research overview of the potential biologic benefits of physical activity and how these may relate to one's philosophic value system. The second part of the book offers a historical-philosophical perspective of the changing role of exercise in the life of man. Parts Three and Four analyze the recently accumulated research evidence relating to the effects of activity on biological efficiency and well-being. What adaptations take place in the heart, lungs, and blood vessels with endurance conditioning? What modifications in the muscle and bone tissue occur during one's participation in a weight-lifting program designed to improve strength? What does research indicate in regard to the most effective methods for stretching the body connective tissue to improve joint range of motion? These are exemplary practical questions for the intellectually curious student who is interested in scientific principles underlying a realistic and intelligent plan of physical activity for adulthood. The last part of the book outlines specific recommendations for the development of scientifically based training programs for strength, flexibility, and endurance. Desirable outcomes of such programs represent potential values to those willing to pay the price.

This book is designed primarily for college men and women enrolled in courses in Physical Fitness, Body Conditioning, Body Mechanics, Adapted Physical Education, or Foundations of Physical Education. The text is adaptable to courses in Health Education, Recreation, Rehabilitation, Physical Medicine and other areas concerned with the values of physical activity in preventive medicine. It may also be appropriately used as a basic reference for any college level physical activity course in which there is concern for the comprehensive carryover values of physical activity in adult life. The historical material could be utilized in courses in History of Physical Education, and Socio-Psychological Foundations of Physical Education. Moreover, and of equal importance, this book should be valuable to any woman or man interested in searching for scientific and philosophic understandings and explanations relative to one's setting up a logical plan for the role of exercise in her or his life mode.

The authors would like to thank Dr. George Q. Rich, III, of the Physical Education Department, and Mr. Saul Bernstein of the Two Dimension Art Department, California State University, Northridge, for their kind assistance in the photography and rendering of the exercise illustrations.

# PART 1

## Planning For Biologic Outcomes of Muscular Activity

**OVERVIEW**   The human organism has an innate biological need for physical activity. The heart, lungs, skeleton, muscles, and nervous system respond qualitatively to the regular stress of exercise. To enjoy maximum benefits of physical activity basic principles of training or conditioning should be adhered to. Application of these principles provides for a regular, balanced, safe program of training which does not place undue demands on the human physiology.

In order to analyze the personal role of physical activity in one's present and future life-style, it is necessary to analyze the philosophic bases of value(s), including biological, cultural, and psychosocial values. It is therefore necessary to understand the kinds and sources of *your* values. If such understandings are gained, they may lead to the incorporation of enjoyable forms of beneficial kinds of physical activity in one's life scheme.

# 1 | Fundamental Biologic Principles of Physical Activity: Scientific Considerations

A SYNTHESIS of the research evidence presented in this text regarding the biological outcomes of physical activity supports the contention that the human organism genetically possesses an innate biological demand or need for the regular stress of exercise. The effect of such activity stress is to improve the functional response of the various physiological systems, with the most dramatic changes taking place in the neuromuscular, skeletal, cardiovascular and pulmonary systems, as well as the oxygen transport mechanism. These improvements in physiological function are the result of biological adaptation or modification to regular exercise stress. Part 3 of the book addresses itself to the major biological adjustments to physical activity. Review of Part 3 will provide the reader with a better understanding of the relationship of physical activity to the biological quantity and quality of life.

The biological adaptations which occur in response to exercise stress and conditioning can provide for significantly improved quality of living (6). Individuals who pursue a regular program of balanced physical activity designed to improve and maintain strength, flexibility (joint range of motion), and cardiorespiratory efficiency (endurance) can engage in much more vigorous and varied recreational pursuits. Such activities as mountain climbing, backpacking, cross-country skiing, and scuba diving are not inappropriate for the healthy adult who maintains a balanced, year-round fitness program. Other adults who do not exercise regularly may be limited to much more sedentary recreational and avocational pursuits which involve spectatorship or light physical activity, such as golf or shuffleboard. The average adult unnecessarily limits his potential for activity with age because of his unwillingness to maintain a regular conditioning program. There are reports of even very elderly individuals who continued to athletically train and perform at remarkably high levels, some in endurance events such as the marathon. There is no research evidence that continued physical activity, even into old age, produces any serious physiological complications, providing of course that reasonable principles of training and conditioning are adhered to by the normal healthy adult. In addition, the fit adult who maintains a high degree of muscular strength and tonus exhibits better postural mechanics and gives visual evidence of a lesser percentage of body fat and a greater percentage of lean body mass. It is well demonstrated that absence of obesity lessens the adult's predisposition for a host of chronic diseases, most importantly the cardiovascular syndromes (5).

Part 4 of the book outlines for the unsophisticated physical education student the biological bases for improved muscular strength, joint range of motion (flexibility) and endurance (cardiorespiratory efficiency). The understandings developed from Part 3 shall provide the scientific basis for establishment of a balanced, individualized physical activity regimen. The student shall understand why as well as how to pursue the three major dimensions of biological fitness.

Only minimal consideration has been given in this book to the considerable sociopsychological values of longitudinal physical activity. The changes in self-image which are incidental to one's improvement in physical fitness have significant implications for positive personality adjustment manifestations. Any person who regularly enjoys the attributes of vigorous activity can describe in his or her own terms the beneficial "feelings" or relief which readily ensue. For this reason it is believed that exercise can serve as a significant psychological medium for the sublimation or relief of tension. Participation in group recreational activities can serve as a significant social outlet. Such benefits are difficult to scientifically document, but in reality may represent one of the most significant personal values of muscular activity for the modern, urban-dwelling female or male.

The woman or man planning to develop a personal physical activity program should follow some established concepts of conditioning which are substantiated by years of research in the human performance exercise physiology laboratory. The applications of these major concepts are outlined later in this chapter, but some of the more general considerations are provided first. These general considerations shall provide a safe practical basis for initial planning of a physical conditioning program while the reader is becoming more familiar with the biological foundations of exercise.

## GENERAL CONSIDERATIONS

*Age.* It is broadly assumed that one's tolerance or capacity for exercise gradually diminishes with increasing age. Although there is general agreement that physical performance shows a decrease with age in the years subsequent to achievement of physiological maturity, the relationship is not clear-cut (2). It is difficult to separate the effect of "disuse" or inactivity upon performance from the more pure physiological or degenerative effects of aging. Maximum strength and maximum work capacity (maximum oxygen consumption) do decrease with the approach of middle and old age. Astrand (1), however, has shown that the mechanical efficiency with which work is performed on the bicycle ergometer is not affected by age.

Practical experience with fitness programs for the middle-aged and elderly suggests that such elements of the population should practice intelligent caution in planning their reconditioning regimen. All adults should have a complete physical examination prior to initiation of activity. This medical examination should include an exercise electrocardiogram. With increasing age the intensity of the training program should be moderated and smaller increments of progression planned for. With an increase in both age and number of years of sedentary living, a greater time span will be required for significant improvement in physiological function. Moreover, individuals who have been very sedentary should avoid "all out" vigorous activity which places undue and acute strain on the heart and blood vessels.

*Sex.* Most references to physical fitness and body conditioning have been directed toward the male. This is unfortunate, since the female stands to achieve the same physiological benefits of training as the male. There is little evidence to support the popular belief that the female's exercise capacity is significantly inferior to that of the male. In fact, analysis of world championship performances indicates that the female achieves 80 to 91 percent of the best male records, this despite the fact that world level athletic competition for women is of comparatively recent origin (3). When remaining cultural inhibitions are eradicated, it is not inconceivable that individual females may surpass the best male performance in selected athletic events. The increasingly higher quality of female swimmers' performance is evidence of such a possibility.

There is no substantial evidence to indicate that the most vigorous of physical activity is significantly detrimental to the female anatomy or physiology. Klaus (5) reports more connective tissue injuries to female than male athletes, but this probably represents structural or morphological tissue differences. There is no basis for the common belief that strenuous activity creates unusual menstrual or gynecological problems (1, 4). One exception to this is a slightly increased susceptibility to vaginal infection among competitive swimmers who train for long periods during the menstrual period. There is conflicting evidence and clinical opinion regarding the effects of menstruation upon the performance of physical activity and vice versa (3). It has been widely recognized that most female athletes do not allow the menstrual cycle to interfere with their performance. It would seem logical, therefore, that much of the female's fear of physical exertion during menstruation is learned. Young girls should be encouraged to seek their highest limits for muscular activity, regardless of the timing of the menstrual cycle, and thus learn to individually moderate their levels of exercise at various times during the cycle. Obviously, during pregnancy the exercise program must be significantly modified in consultation with the obstetrician. During and after pregnancy, special consideration should be given to maintenance of abdominal muscle strength and tonus.

*Motivation.* Perhaps no other factor accounts for the success or failure of a reconditioning program more than psychological motivation. To foster continued motivation in a conditioning program it is important to make exercising fun. Thus, the goal of achieving a sufficient level of conditioning to permit safe participation in dual and team sports such as tennis, volleyball and basketball is recommended. In this way, conditioning activities can be pursued which offer variety and the additional opportunity for socialization with other people. The very unfit adult, however, must avoid competition early in his reconditioning program so as to avoid overextending himself. Also, the conditioning program should be conducted in a pleasant physical environment, outdoors if possible. Joggers should use the local park or school facility where they can run on the grass and so avoid the common and depressing problem of foot strain and shin splints.

Physical fitness motivation is also dependent upon knowledge of improvement or progress. Therefore, it is advisable to chart body weight changes, resting and recovery heart rate and strength performances, as well as running, swimming or bicycling progress which would serve to demonstrate the efficacy of the training effect. Also, it should be emphasized that a reasonable progression be established that will not become a drudgery and thus curtail enthusiasm and motivation.

Lastly, attention should be given to proper rest and diet so that adequate physiological reserve will be maintained. Probably there will be a slightly increased demand for longer sleep periods. The diet requires no special modification, provided a balanced complement of fats, proteins and carbohydrates, with emphasis on the latter, is eaten on a regular daily basis. Meals should number no fewer than two per day so that adequate blood sugar levels are maintained for the exercise period. Daily caloric intake should not be increased if you are attempting to reduce body weight. Careful attention to the above factors will significantly assist in maintaining optimum motivation during the early weeks and months of a reconditioning program. After several months of perseverance the program of activities becomes part of one's daily life pattern and the individual will find himself looking forward to it and missing it when unable to exercise. Part of this motivational change is a reflection of the physiochemical adaptations of the human body's response to muscular activity and is related to the organism's innate biological demand for movement stress. These adaptations are outlined in rather complete fashion in Part 3 of the book.

**APPLICATIONS**

*Balance.*   In developing the individual fitness program primary consideration should be given to inclusion of activities which stimulate the improvement of muscular strength, endurance and flexibility. Muscular strength is important for maintaining good postural mechanics and firm muscles, whereas flexibility is necessary for the prevention of connective tissue injury and neuromuscular syndromes related to shortening of the tissue. Of these three aspects of fitness cardiorespiratory endurance is undoubtedly the most important and should be given the largest proportion of time in your program by way of running, cycling, swimming or related endurance activity. Chapter 10 provides more specific recommendations for the development and maintenance of endurance factors.

*Specificity.*   It shall be apparent from the discussions in the fourth section of this book that the biological adaptations to conditioning or training stimuli are highly specific. This is why special techniques for the development of strength, flexibility and endurance are outlined in Chapters 8, 9, and 10. It is most appropriate to begin the daily conditioning program with specific stretching activities, followed by calisthenic type activities for muscle tonus and strength. Later, light weights may be used several times per week for optimum strength development. The latter part of the daily workout should stress cardiorespiratory endurance activities of at least 10–15 minutes duration.

Another important application of the specificity concept is its implication relative to personal variations in sports or recreational participation. Because of the specialized response of the connective tissue and physiological systems to training, it is possible to be very fit for certain vigorous activities and not for others. Therefore, one should gradually train for and participate in the activities which he wishes to pursue recreationally. The individual might, for example, be very fit for playing handball but become very fatigued and subsequently suffer from post-exercise physiological distress and connective tissue soreness when participating in another vigorous sport such as basketball. The female might be very fit for playing badminton but fatigue very quickly the first time she participates in modern dance activities. Or the individual connective tissue might be well adapted to running on a grass surface but become very irritated and sore when an attempt is made to run on a concrete or asphalt surface. Middle-aged and older persons should particularly avoid participating in activities for which they have not specifically trained because of the unusual and acute stress it places upon the systemic physiology and structural tissue, such as bone, ligaments, tendons, and so on.

*Regularity.* Some regular program of conditioning must be established in order for the participant to be able to appreciate significant improvement in strength, endurance and flexibility. Practical results from various fitness training programs have generally demonstrated that a minimum of three days per week must be devoted to the conditioning endeavor. More optimum results can be obtained from a five-day-per-week program. Ideally, the recreational-fitness program should be initiated in adolescence or early adulthood and followed throughout life. In this way the biological systems are not irregularly acutely stressed through the medium of exercise.

When training weights are being used to stimulate strength development it is not necessary to train in this fitness dimension more than three or even two days per week. (See Chapter 8.) Endurance activities should be pursued at least three days per week and preferably more often. Flexibility stretching activities require very little time and can be conducted on a daily basis. (See Chapter 9.) A reasonable approach is to pursue strength predominately on a 2–3-day-per-week basis and endurance predominately on a 3–4-day-per-week basis. On each day the strength or endurance activity is preceded by flexibility stretching.

The time of day reserved for the conditioning activities is not significant, although it should be a time that does not require rushing, so that the experience is regularly an enjoyable one. Also, the period immediately after meals should be avoided. Early morning, before breakfast, is usually a practical time for most persons since the energy and motivation level is high, the stomach is empty and there are no other impingements on the person's time and motivation. In this way, it is less likely that other responsibilities will interfere with the conduct of the training program.

*Warm-Up.* Each conditioning session should adhere to this concept. Ideally, any vigorous activity should be preceded by 5–10 minutes of stretching for all the major muscles and related connective tissue. Then, very gradual increases in the work load for strength or endurance improvement should be applied. In this way, the early part of the workout calls for very low energy expenditure, with the intensity and duration of the work bout being gradually increased. For example, in a jogging endurance regimen, walking or alternate walking-running would constitute at least the first five minutes of the program, followed by more vigorous running near the middle of the workout. As pointed out in Chapter 10, fifteen minutes of warm-up is probably more beneficial for the older adult. In this way, the imposition of sudden extreme stress upon the heart, blood vessels and other organs and physiological systems is avoided. The latter part of the workout period is devoted to physiologically "cooling down," i.e., gradually deaccelerating the level of energy output. At least five minutes of very easy running followed by a period of continued walking insures that pulmonary, cardiovascular and metabolic function can *gradually* return to the resting or basal level. The warm up and cool down concept is most important in its application to any endurance conditioning program and is critically important for the middle-aged or older adult who might be susceptible to cardiovascular disorder. In addition, it should be remembered that careful and prolonged warm up will help to minimize the possibility of connective tissue injury during vigorous activity. More information on this biological relationship is given in Chapter 9.

*Overload.* This concept implies that for significant improvement in any aspect of conditioning the appropriate physiological systems have to be overloaded, that is to say, stressed at a level beyond that to which they are normally stressed. In Chapter 8 consideration is given to the application of this concept to strength development through gradual increase of the resistance increments from week to week so as to progressively and safely overload the neuromuscular system and connective tissue. The concept applies equally to flexibility stretching routines in which the elastic tissue is progressively mechanically elongated so as to increase range of joint motion. After many months and years of such progressive overload, gymnasts and modern dancers are able to achieve remarkable flexibility in specific joints.

As pointed out in Chapter 10, endurance training programs make effective use of overload upon the entire oxygen transport mechanism (lungs, heart, and blood vessels) by modifying the intensity or duration of the endurance training stimulus. Use of the interval training concept permits significant overload of the $O_2$ transport system. Short vigorous repetitive bouts of swimming, running or cycling are used to stimulate the high metabolic energy output. Short rest periods are used between interval endurance bouts. Physiologically, endurance overload can be increased by: (1) increasing the intensity of the work bout (higher energy output by swimming, running or bicycling faster), (2) increasing the duration of each bout (such as from forty to sixty seconds), (3) increasing the number of interval bouts at each training session (such as from 5 to 7) or (4) decreasing the rest period between interval bouts (as from 1½ minutes to 1 minute). When progressive overload results in the *desired* level of strength, endurance or flexibility, further modification (overload) of the training stimulus is not required and a maintenance program may be followed.

*Maintenance.* A maintenance program is that program followed for the continuation of a given achieved level of strength, endurance or flexibility. Obviously then, the maintenance training stimulus involves no additional overload. Such a program, designed to sustain achieved levels of fitness rather than to stimulate further improvement, utilizes a static training stimulus—no further increase in resistance for strength, no further increase in the intensity or duration of the endurance training stimulus, and no further increase in the mechanical stretch stimulus for flexibility. When one has achieved what is a practical level of fitness or conditioning, obviously no such further increases in the training variable are necessary.

Fortunately, a maintenance program is more comfortable and easy to sustain than a progressive overload training program. When the point reached in a conditioning program permits implementation of the maintenance concept, it is much less difficult to train at each session and thus one appreciates a higher level of motivation and enjoyment. In other words, it is much less physiologically stressful to pursue a maintenance program than it is a progressive overload training program. Unfortunately, lack of knowledge of this fact allows many persons to quit a reconditioning program before they reach this facilatory level of maintenance. Part 4 directs attention to the specific biologic applications of the maintenance principle to strength, endurance and flexibility.

Recognition should be accorded the fact that a period of voluntary or forced inactivity (e.g., illness or injury) results in a loss of the physiological training effect. This so-called "detraining effect" is proportionate to the training effect, which is to say that the beneficial physiological effects of a strength, endurance or flexibility training program are lost during detraining at about the same rate that they were gained. Stated another way the detraining curve is approximately equal to the training curve. For example, if it took six weeks to improve your time in the mile run by 30 seconds, this improvement would be lost during about six weeks of detraining or deconditioning. Thus, whenever it becomes necessary to curtail training for a short period of time during a regimen of maintenance it requires the reapplication of an overload training stimulus in order to regain the original qualitative level of physiological efficiency.

When an individual decides to temporarily suspend a maintenance or conditioning program, detraining should be planned on a very gradual basis. If several months of training were required to achieve a given level of strength, endurance or flexibility then about the same period of time should be used to taper off or detrain. In appropriate detraining, the intensity and duration of the training stimuli are gradually reduced, allowing the biologic adaptations of training to diminish slowly.

*Acclimation.* The physical environment in which one trains has profound implications for the efficiency of physiological response. Thus, high heat and humidity should be avoided by choosing the appropriate time of day. Older persons and females should particularly avoid these environmental stress conditions since their heat tolerance is somewhat lower. Clothing should be light and loose fitting so as to provide good cutaneous (surface) circulation and ventilation for evaporative cooling of the sweat. Also, days during which high air pollution concentrations are present should be avoided, although early morning training in the urban setting usually precludes this problem.

When it becomes necessary to change one's geographical locale and climate it will take several weeks for the various physiological systems to efficiently adapt to the change of environment during exercise stress. Thus, moving from a moderate climate at sea level to higher altitude or a hot climate will require a period of time for biological adaptation or acclimation. You should not expect to perform as well in your conditioning activities in the new clime as you did previously. The period of time for physiological acclimation to occur will vary with one's age and the degree of environmental change involved in the geographic relocation.

## SUMMARY

Man has an innate biological, social, and psychological instinct and need for physical activity. Regular participation in exercise is related to both the quantity and quality of life. General and specific biological adaptations occur during man's participation in programs designed to improve strength, endurance and flexibility. A review of the research literature provides practical biological principles for the development of safe, efficient and balanced conditioning programs. To provide for continuity and regularity of physical activity each individual must examine the relationship of the biological values and principles to his personal life-style and philosophy.

## REFERENCES

1. Astrand, P. O. "Aerobic Work Capacity in Men and Women with Special Reference to Age." *Acta Physiolog Scand* 49 (1960) : Suppl. 169.
2. Bortz, E. L. "Exercise, Fitness, and Aging." In *Exercise and Fitness, Q Symposium.* Chicago: Athletic Institute, 1960.
3. deVries, H. *Physiology of Exercise for Physical Education and Athletics.* Dubuque, Iowa: Wm. C. Brown Company, 1974.
4. Erdelyi, G. J. "Gynecological Survey of Female Athletes." *Journal of Sports Medicine* 2 (1962) :174.
5. Klaus, E. J. "The Athletic Status of Women." In *International Research in Sport and Physical Education,* edited by E. Jokl and E. Simon. Springfield, Ill.: Charles C Thomas, 1964.
6. Raab, Wilhelm. *Prevention of Ischemic Heart Disease, Principles and Practices,* Springfield, Ill.: Charles C Thomas, 1966.

# 2 | Personal Values of Physical Activity: Philosophic Considerations

HUMAN BEINGS have always had values. In all times and places, however, they did not identify and select their own personal values. Some of early man's offspring might have been vaguely aware of the impact of value on behavior. If the child or youth of Homo sapiens felt free (momentarily) to express personal choices and preferences, his or her resulting behavior sometimes was in conflict with local mores and customs. Conflicts between social-societal values on the one hand, and individual-personal values on the other, is by no means only a modern-day phenomenon.

Today, a good many children and adolescents seem to be permitted to act in terms of their respective personal values. Many of these adolescents, and in addition, post-adolescents, often prefer to avoid the consequences of superficially selected personal values. They are alert to the difficulty of deciding, among a myriad possible values, which ones to identify as theirs. They recognize the power personal values have in deciding their respective styles of living, as worded by Plato, "life-style."

A major facet of this current philosophic recognition of responsibility in deciding one's life-style and values-selection is represented by the large segment of the population engaging in various forms of physical activity —exercise, sports, the dance, active recreational pursuits, rehabilitative-adaptive-corrective activities, aquatics and boating, winter activities, to name but a few. Apparently, many millions of persons in many nations place value on the outcomes of physical activity other than manual labor.

### THE MEANING OF VALUE(S)

The term "value(s)" in these pages is interpreted to mean that property that indicates a something (object, experience, event, and the like) is wanted or desired by, matters or is important to one or more persons because it is judged good or worthwhile, or is considered to be a Good. Such an interpretation may be viewed by the professional philosopher and axiologist as a rank simplication. The technical philosophic view is far more intricate and vague. With that acknowledgement, and for lack of a more meaningful term, this commonplace interpretation of "value(s)" will be applied when some of the outcomes of physical activity are considered as being potential values, or as having potential value.

Strength and endurance are obvious outcomes of some forms of physical activity. Early man must have come to regard such possessions as desirable and wanted. They mattered to him. Negatively, he must have been aware of their importance as he observed the survival liability of the clumsy, weak, slow and easily-fatigued in tribal life. Positively, he may have had pleasant inner feelings as his superior strength struck the winning blow, as his prowess won the chieftain's seat, or as he ran a formidable distance to warn the tribal settlement, in time, of the approaching enemy. Such a conjecture seems to be of interest for a reason other than its historical possibility. Regardless of one's cultural sophistication or intellectual brilliance, human living is significantly influenced by human judgment of that which is regarded as a value, or to be of value.

As tribes coalesced into nations, as the Age of Individual Betterment, the Epoch of Social and Cultural Growth and Development, and the Era of National Preservation followed, the values engendered by engaging in physical activity increased in number, kind and significance. That extension and augmentation emerged slowly. But as educators and researchers, scientists and philosophers unified and directed their efforts and thought, the expansion and enriching of concepts of value rapidly accelerated. Chapters 3 and 4 undertake a review of that transition.

### KINDS OF VALUE(S)

It is not unusual for consideration of personal values to lead into thinking about social values. Most humans accept and possess social values. They also choose to live within the limitations which societal values place on them. Nor are there impregnable walls surrounding these different kinds of value, as the names might imply. Like other kinds of value, they spill over and seep through such language barriers, although the names do facilitate analysis, identification and better understanding.

Such values as cooperation; membership in a group; losing with good grace and winning without pretense; and, ethical-moral responsibility are related in some ways with: respect for the rights of others; considering the safety of others; providing for alternating leadership and followership; sportsmanship; adjusting to the give and take of the game; fair play; friendliness; taking praise and blame with equanimity; and, respect for the rules. Emotional control, honesty and truthfulness although heavy with social connotations are easily regarded as individual values.

Societal-cultural values also are seen as related to those just mentioned. Here are a few examples taken from those formulated for this country by three different nationwide committees (2, 3, 4) of social anthropologists, cosmologists, scientists, philosophers and historians: (1) central concern for the individual; (2) leisure for worthy ends; (3) ethical and moral action; (4) integral relationships with others; and (5) appreciation and production of the aesthetic. These may be considered as societal-cultural values, and also as those one may seek, having some large-scale values for national programs of physical education and recreation(1).

Possible regrettable results of presenting lists similar to those in the two previous paragraphs are, on the one hand, the reader instantly accepting them without self-application, and on the other hand, his possible rejection of them as merely fine-sounding statements of the hyprocrite. Those who take this latter stance, with justification, should continue to express it. Although the "hyprocrite" may have good intentions, he or she may gain from being sharply reminded that agreeing with a Good, symbolized by a word or two, without self-application, is one of the easiest things to do.

Another difficult-to-catergorize kind of value is the absolute-relative complex. The prime purpose of these paragraphs is to preclude any exploration of the long-discussed issue, absolutism vs relativism. It is suggested that unless one happens to have "the answers," he might feel richly repaid if she or he *studies* both views without bias. That suggestion does not prevent one comment before turning to another kind of value. Some persons regard Good, Truth, Justice and Beauty as *the* four absolute values. Should they be such, are there not some easy-to-find outcomes of participation in physical activities that may be linked with these four master values?

Most types of the dance are generally associated with aesthetics and thus with Beauty. Many biologic values, when properly conducted, contribute to mankind's good and thus to Good. Truth and Justice challenge the athlete, the coach and those responsible for the conduct of sport. Amos Alonzo Stagg is this century's classic example of one who aspired to meet that challenge. Though there be few today who resemble him in this respect, the potentiality and the opportunity still exist. It continues to be remarkable how the example set by one individual may stimulate great accomplishments by those on whom he has had a more than passing influence.

One professor of a college graduate course dealing with personal values was curious about what modern young adults believed were absolute values. The effort continued for more than two decades. Rather consistently, the following were mentioned more frequently: Life, Happiness, Human Personality and the Creator. Even here the outcomes of some physical activities seem to point to some of these values.

Another "either-or" kind of value is the objective-subjective dualism. Such biologic values as flexibility and cardiorespiratory efficiency are regarded as objective, while enjoyment, exultation and courage are subjective values. As indicated above, categorization is less clean-cut than is sometimes indicated. For example, in order to attain personal well-being (a complex of objective and subjective values) certain outcomes must be forthcoming. Should the individual fail to acquire the desired well-being, despair, discouragement, despondency and other subjective disvalues may result. However, as strength, cardiorespiratory efficiency and some other objectively valued outcomes are acquired, steps then may be taken to continue toward attaining well-being, provided a subjective value, perseverance, supported by the individual's *Will*, is effectively applied.

### SOME SOURCES OF VALUE(S)

The self-asked question, "From where do my personal values come?" is ever available to anyone intent upon formulating the best possible life style for herself or himself. Each adult—regardless of chronological age —may experience situations in which he or she thinks of selection of personal values as unique, original and the result of solely his or her own ideas. In a sense, this may be. Nevertheless, the *roots* of values are almost always multifold. For example, here are some rather common sources: (1) current subjective experiences in general; (2) current aesthetic experiences in particular; (3) influences of contemporaries; (4) genetic heritage; (5) influences of family, state, church, school, and communication media; (6) one's reasoning ability; (7) past experiences not covered in the foregoing; (8) one's feelings about and attitudes toward each and all of the foregoing; and (9) the creation of possible and actual new ideas. Some persons prefer to believe that all things good come from the Creator. Others insist that all values are products of their own minds.

The effort to ferret out and reason through the source(s) of any value which is being considered usually pays off. Should an objective outcome of physical activities such as cardiorespiratory efficiency prove to be of value most persons would regard it more favorably than if the source were one's unsupported opinion. One of the advantages of values emerging from participating in physical activity is that many of those values can be supported with respectable researches. On the other hand, this does not mean that values lacking scientific support are to be held suspect or to be belittled or ignored. Those values relating to outcomes which are observable but immeasurable, such as respect for the rights of others, may be as desirable as a scientifically-measurable outcome such as muscular strength. And some values, because of the nature of the related outcomes rest, at least in part, on the experience of the human race. Outcomes that emerge from current subjective experiences in general, if this is the most dependable medium, still may be of value. Obviously, the key to this situation is that one makes as certain as conditions permit to find the best possible source(s) for each value under consideration.

One reason for placing emphasis on the examination of sources of one's selection of values is that the process of deciding is fraught with such possible weaknesses as the following: (1) lack of satisfactory guides; (2) unsupported personal opinion; (3) uncertain criteria for personal judgments; (4) inadequacy of the counseling of some contemporaries; (5) personal inexperience in value-selection; (6) shrugging off responsibility for consequences of one's decision; and (7) overconfidence or underconfidence in one's ability to make value decision. The inexperienced selector of personal values can take heart, however. No human being so far has been born with expert judgment in these matters. All who have gone before him as well as many of his contemporaries have found the task difficult, vexing, uncertain, and continual. But, the weight of these disvalues is lightened by knowing where a considered value's sources are, and by knowing which of those sources are most dependable.

### SELECTING PHYSICAL ACTIVITIES OF PERSONAL VALUE

Gaining confidence in the reliability of one's judgment of and decisions regarding personal values, as one considers engaging in physical activity, usually is a long drawn-out process. This process may be shortened considerably, although the following steps at first glance seem to refute that statement.

There seem to be, within the reach of almost anyone, many excuses for not participating in physical activities. Although there are of course some fully valid reasons, in addition there are some ridiculously flimsy ones. Yet, millions of youth and adults, despite their novice status, demonstrate preferences for engaging in physical activity and thus gaining attendant values, by making the effort, devoting the time and expending the energy.

How does one coordinate his or her personal values with physical activities?

Here are some suggested steps:

1. Jot down on a sheet of paper those various aspects of life which encompass the ingredients of your life. Here are some examples: home, school, church, health, happiness, government, social relationships, organic vigor, leisure, freedom, aesthetics, success, personality, ethic-morals, avocations and vocation. Do not be bothered by various "sizes" of these aspects of life.

2. Rank the aspects you have selected in order of importance, as they apply to your life-style. You can add to this original list later on.

3. Opposite each aspect jot down *kinds* of values you feel may be involved in that aspect. For example, opposite "school" would be individual, social and cultural values (in addition to possible others).

4. Now rank the *kinds* of values you have listed, according to the number of times each kind has been listed. If this ranking does not roughly agree with your prior judgment of which *kinds* of values are most important to you, reconsider your ranking and revise if necessary.

5. Now, check all the *kinds* of values you have listed to make sure as possible that all your personal values can be covered later on. Also, add or delete any aspects of life which will make that list more accurate.

6. For *each* of your top-ranking *kinds* of values (roughly, the top 50 percent) formulate concise, sound reasons why you believe it "deserves" a high ranking. Then, do the same thing for the lowest ranking values (why are they *values* even though they are ranked at the bottom?)

7. Now, for *each* top-ranking *kind* of value, make a list of its subsidiary values. For example, for the biologic kind of value, you might list such a value as muscular strength, muscular endurance, and so on. Number these subsidiary values so that the most important one is No. 1 and so on down to the least important for each *kind* of value.

8. Examine all of these lists of subsidiary values in order to see if

each value is ranked approximately where it belongs in terms of your intended life style.

9. Now, consider all of the subsidiary values, *regardless* of the *kind* of values which encompass it, and rank them all in a master list of your values. For example, suppose you ranked Biological Values as third in your list of *kinds* of values. And, suppose you have listed as one of its subsidiary values, cardiorespiratory efficiency. But, now that you look at *all* subsidiary values together, you are convinced that this value is one of the *most* important of all values. So, this ranking results in a more accurate list of your personal values, regardless of its category of "kind."

10. Now, consider all of the different forms of physical activity which you like as a participant and those in which you might be interested as a participant. As you look at your ranking of values, and look at the physical activities you prefer, which of the latter are most promising as potential sources of your most important values? Are there, then, some of your top values which could come to the fore to be achieved if you extended your list of physical activities? Which are those activities?

In order to provide some bases for further examining your most favored values, a "Ten-Point Test of Values" is helpful. Submit each of your top-ranking values to each of the following questions:

a. How "large" is this value? Covers what?
b. What is its source(s)? What of the source's quality?
c. How flexible or rigid is this value?
d. Does it lead to other values, potentially?
e. If conditions change, can the value adjust and adapt?
f. Is it stable or weakly founded? Easily eradicated?
g. Does this value consider the rights of others?
h. How strongly do you plan to retain this value?
i. Does its realization depend on difficult-to-control factors?
j. What important (to you) purposes does this value serve?

One cannot be too careful in the selection of personal values in fashioning one's life-style, so important are they. As participation in physical activities is considered, here are some questions which might well be answered by the individual: (1) Is this a value which is popular among your friends? (2) How does it compare with others of your values as to its essentiality? (3) What conditions or situations would probably influence you to jettison this value? (4) What does this value have to do with the betterment of your status—with your acquiring the life-style you presently prefer? (5) What are the costs of maintaining this as a value (time, effort, energy, thought, possibly money)?

In selecting physical activities which "match" the values one has selected, such principles as the following might well be followed:

a. Obtain clearance from a licensed physician or other adequately qualified professional, if you have been sedentary for several months.
b. Begin slowly and easily even if you have been sedentary for only a month or two.
c. If advisable, select at least one activity which provides a vigorous workout, if time is an important factor.
d. Select at least one activity that provides a moderate workout in a moderate amount of time.
e. Select one activity which offsets ill-effects of vocationally-oriented body positions (dentist, barber, stenographer, and so on).
f. Formulate an overall program geared to your physical condition and the provisions of the local environment.
g. If feasible, build a program that is enjoyable and variable.

### SUMMARY

Mathematical values stem from antiquity. Economic values are centuries old. Philosophic values, as properties, are timeless; as *named* properties, they are about two hundred years old.

The outcomes of engaging in physical activity under suitable conditions have been regarded as humanly beneficial to and for the individual since he and she became thinking man and woman. They have been considered to be values, or of value, as the individual (or as the social order) wants or desires them, and, because they matter and are important to him or her.

There are a number of different kinds of values—biological, cultural, psychosocial, and so on. A good many personal values may be realized at least in part by means of participation in physical activity. The worth of personal values is significantly dependent on their sources. The individual who wishes to avoid shallow selections of values for his life-style should *examine* not only his values but the quality of their sources.

In the interest of presenting aids to avoid this shallowness, a number of devices have been submitted. In spite of the time which this examining and re-examining requires of the individual, it nevertheless short-cuts the achievement of reliability in one's judgment of and decisions regarding the values which he seeks in physical activity.

## REFERENCES

1. Allen, Catherine L.; Davis, E. C.; Lynn, Minnie L.; and Wallis, Earl. Report of the President's Committee on "The Significance of the Profession in American Culture." *Journal of Health, Physical Education, Recreation.* November-December 1964, pp. 37–43.

2. *Goals for Americans.* Englewood Cliffs, N.J.: Prentice-Hall, 1964.

3. Jessup, John K. et al. *The National Purpose.* New York: Holt, Rinehart & Winston, 1960.

4. Morison, Elting Elmore. *The American Style.* New York: Harper & Brothers, 1958.

# PART 2

## Historic and Philosophic Foundations of Biologic Values

**OVERVIEW**    Aside from his cunning and emotions, early man would not have survived without the beneficial outcomes of his physical activity. Without knowing about values as such, our early forebears placed value upon these outcomes. The very presence of the weak, clumsy, easily fatigued and slow could have left no doubt about the desirability of their opposites.

With the coming of early nations and the division of labor, each category of human activity—manual laborer, house-keeper, soldier, craftsman, physician-priest, scribe and royalty —learned the value of the outcomes of its physical activities in its life-style.

What yesterday's man and woman *did* with their genetic heritage and with their environment resulted in some changes. Yet, some outcomes remained as legacies to today's man and woman. A great many modern kinds of physical activity, together with their biological values began in antiquity. Certainly, most American sports, exercise and the dance stem from European precursors. In turn, most European specifics in physical activity slowly emerged from the ancient Greeks.

As the early tribesman's hunch and guess joined with the modern scientist's findings, there emerged a great many biological values suggestive of choices for one's personal system of values.

# 3 | Physical Activity Values and Man's Heritage

MODERN MAN engaging in physical activities, like his hoary ancestor, expects outcomes that are beneficial to him if certain conditions are met. Some such fleeting ideas as, "It is good to move vigorously," or, "Exercise is good for you," eventually became a vague sort of maxim. But, as with many other items of folklore, scientists continue to find facts in support of these ideas. Some of the resultants of participating in muscular activity are labeled psychosocial. Some, biological. The latter kinds of outcomes are the center of, but not the sole concern of this book, in acknowledgment of man's unity.

It seems a reasonable guess that pre- and early man began and continued to count on favorable, personal consequences of being physically active, although he probably failed to identify or connect either the cause or the effect. He felt good. He felt tired. He felt exulted. He felt exhausted. Eventually, he must have connected such feelings with his physical efforts. Still later, the relationship between certain kinds of efforts and, say, increased strength, must have been noticed.

Modern researchers in such fields as biochemistry, medicine, physiology and physical education continue, from year to year, to report findings indicating additional, favorable biophysical results to the participant in sports, exercise, vigorous outdoor life, the dance and manual labor. Even the man-in-the-street, whose scope of reading may not exceed today's headlines, is reminded often enough that scientifically-determined facts support the time-crusted maxim. If perchance he is a selective reader he learns of new instrumentation for and new conditions governing the measurement of related parameters.

Before considering these more recent, related findings, let us examine briefly some of the highlights of man's experiences as he gradually began to use and then to plan physical activities as a means of indirectly and unconsciously, then directly and consciously, gaining and retaining biological values. Chapters 4 and 5 also serve as an historic-philosophic introduction to five chapters which present and discuss the major biological values of muscular activity together with their respective main supporting, scientifically-determined facts.

### SURVIVAL

As one conjectures about pre- and early man, one has the impression that few of our progenitors escaped the challenge to survive and the costs of remaining alive. These costs have become increasingly apparent to the anthropologist, the historian of pre-classical antiquity, and the archaeologist, as hard evidence has supplemented conjecturing. Such situations as the following are indicative:

1. There were the demands of trying to gain a livelihood—meeting the rigors of existence—adapting to differing seasons, locations and climates with resulting requirements of shelter, clothing and food paralleled by the building of dwellings, boats and sleds, and the need to hunt, fish and trap, and to gather, prepare and store food.

2. The presence or likelihood of human enemies demanded the development, use and improvement of the tools and skills of scouting, fighting, weaponry and protective devices, flanked by strength, endurance, hardihood, and mind-sets evolving from dances, religio-military activities, and the antics of the shaman or physician-priest.

3. The proximity of wild animals, both a threat to life and a challenge to domestic-militaristic usage, led to such activities as trapping, caging, tethering, corraling, taming and training them, fighting them—or flight. The distances run and walked could have been incredible.

4. Man contended with the "great senseless forces" such as floods, snow, earthquakes, fog, ice, prairie and forest fires, lightning, hail, rain, tidal waves, hurricanes, typhoons, excessive heat, cold and wind. Such forces were among man's greatest fears not only because of their unpredictability, variety and multiplicity, but also because of their vicious impact and his inability and resultant failure to concoct ways to anticipate, meet or counter them. To this day many of these forces have not been

tamed. Certainly they posed different kinds of physical effort by early man. It is little wonder he sought to deal with them by using nonphysical as well as physical techniques.

5. In placating, worshipping, honoring and sacrificing to the gods, man engaged in such activities as the dance, festivals, ceremonials, rituals, and even in Homer's day, sports.

6. Using, demonstrating, displaying, competing in and testing physical prowess in familial and tribal affairs must have occupied some of man's time.

7. Playing; trying-out, idly dabbling, "experimenting" with familiar as well as new ways of performing physical activities and techniques would have been indulged in during times of leisure.

8. Man had to perform home-centered chores (including some of the physical activities mentioned above) such as: tilling the soil, planting, water-carrying, harvesting, food-gathering-storing-preparing, fire-building, wood-gathering, laundering, irrigating, caring for and training animals.

9. He used and developed crafts such as leather-work, weaving various materials, metal-work, wood-work, stone-work, weapon-making and repairing, and the making of clothing.

10. Man also engaged in creative-artistic activities such as cave-drawings, totem-pole making, making and decorating pottery objects, tile, iron, clothing, jewelry, sculptures, utensils, stele and body-decoration.

11. He moved home-sites, which included packing, carrying, walking, hauling, boat-loading, rowing/paddling, rafting, sledding, pushing and pulling.

This detailing of some of the situations met by many members of groups of early mankind with some suggestions of his and her related physical activities present a partial view at best. To say that during many waking hours they must have been physically active seems a reasonable assumption. Although an old saying omitted a crucial concept or two, it was descriptive, for as man is viewed from afar, he "was what he was because of what he and the human race did." Most of the "doing" was of a physical nature.

And, as he did and tried to do an increasing number and variety of things, he learned. One important facet of learning was that of meeting such situations, as outlined above, more effectively—more skillfully and efficiently. He also stumbled onto new ways. He "invented" new ways. He gradually learned to be more self-observant. He learned to be aware of the need for certain kinds of strength, endurance, quickness, steadiness, accuracy, speed and physical toughness, as he met or failed to meet certain conditions, circumstances and challenges.

Eventually, he learned how important it was to the life and survival of family and tribe that as many members as feasible come to possess certain physical attributes. It is therefore not unexpected that chieftains and tribal leaders are portrayed as physically superior men, even though some of them are known to have also played the roles of physician, priest, or shaman.

Eventually, well-led, strong tribes conquered smaller, weaker tribes, which resulted in still larger social units covering greater areas of land and perhaps such assets as rivers, trade-routes and mineral sites. Cultural anthropologists consider the discovery of an effective process of iron-making, together with the spreading of this knowledge and know-how, had a very favorable impact not only on agriculture and industry but also on the military. The implications are clear for the starting of early nations and civilization itself even though the balances of power shifted from time to time.

With such developments, the individual's major responsibility shifted from a familial/tribal focus to that of serving the "state." As new ideas arose and levels of existence changed, the individual's old biological competencies and resources were no longer crucial. The division-of-labor concept and practice arose and were accentuated and extended. This enabled man to expect and receive personal and familial security even though concepts of self and family changed. Organizing many of mankind on the basis of nations brought many, deep, and vast changes in and to the individual. He adjusted—eventually at least.

As much as we humans might like to think of our early progenitors as adapting easily and rather quickly, it probably was an excruciatingly slow process—if in fact it has yet been accomplished. However, with the advent of early nations and organized government, the evidence of what man and woman *did* became more available and dependable. Let us briefly glance at them as they engage in muscular activity roughly from the third millennium B.C. to and including the Roman Empire at her ascendancy.

Although separated by thousands of miles, in some instances, early nations showed a good many commonalities in roles and kinds of physical activity engaged in by their respective peoples. Evidence for that statement comes from such sources as: pictographs, sculptings, engravings, carvings, hieroglyphics, drawings, and paintings on tombs, vases, pyramid inner walls, stone tablets, papyrus leaves, pillars, metal and stone slabs, caves, hillsides, rocks, cliffs, stele and jewelry. There are objects connected with agriculture, trade, commerce, household activities and military operations that also offer evidence. As future archaeological "digs" and anthropological sites are increased in number, and techniques improved, additional hard evidence can be expected to show that men and women participated in still other kinds of physical activity.

As indicated above, one of the accompaniments of the rise of early nations was the enlargement of the concept and practice of the division of labor. To the slaves and those without requisite skills went the tasks of hard manual labor from sunup to sundown. The women-folk from such families also performed the household work in the homes of wealthy landowners, royalty, and later, the well-to-do merchant class. Thus, most adults and youth of the slave and peasant class got their physical activity through hard work.

A *second* classification included men in the nation's military services. Their physical activity (in times of peace) consisted of practicing javelin and spear throwing, use of the shield, swordsmanship, firebrand-throwing, horsemanship, slinging, rolling large rocks, archery from foot, horseback or chariot, hunting activities, rowing, sailing, ship-boarding, ship-beaching, repair and care of war paraphernalia including personal equipment.

A *third* group consisted of the artisans and craftsmen. The performance of their vocations provided their principal physical activity. A list of some of the categories in this group indicates that the physical efforts of some were not to be compared in vigor and duration with those of the two groups just mentioned. Some of these men were stone masons, carpenters, metal workers, manufacturers of iron, brass and bronze objects, silversmiths and goldsmiths, potters, builders, architects, sculptors, painters, musicians, frescoers, leather workers, shipbuilders, makers and repairers of oars, sails and ship's gear. Anthropologists conjecture that some of the products were regarded so highly that the men who made them were specially regarded and worked with the priests and shamans.

These latter together with scribes, draftsmen, notaries, archivists, members of the legal profession, physicians, and royalty constituted a *fourth* group whose physical activity came from outside their vocational activities. If the members of the wealthy class are included here, it is believed that their children attended school and that there, or through private lessons, learned some one or several of the following: the dance, water-centered activities, children's plays and games, and, for the boys particularly, wrestling, archery, equitation, simulated war activities or military-oriented contests and drills, weight-lifting, boxing, and horse-related activities.

It is not astonishing that the dance was among the most ubiquitous physical activities among such early nations as Sumer, Egypt, Babylonia, Mesopotamia, Akkad, Ur, China, India and Persia, as well as the city states of Greece. The Egyptian dances—religious, war, acrobatic, entertainment and folk—are matched by those of China—shield, plume, lance, and flute. Water-centered activities also would be expected in almost all of these early nations—sailing, rowing, swimming, fishing, diving, paddling and boating for pleasure, transportation and naval operations.

In Persia under King Cyrus in the sixth century B.C., the first recorded training of an army by means of athletic sports is found. Van Dalen and Sasajima (4), in *Quest*, report that in China's Chou dynasty (1122–249 B.C.) the well-organized schools emphasized the physical together with the moral, intellectual and aesthetic. The physical emphasis included ceremonial dances and sports as integral parts of formal education. Four different kinds of Chinese football are mentioned by the historians.

According to Kramer (3), eminent American Sumerologist, the first schools were located in Sumer (a number of "textbooks" dating from 2500 B.C. have been excavated). Although the "curriculum" is outlined, no mention is made of any physical activities. And, of Sumer's twenty-seven "firsts" among nations, the only reference (among the translations thus far) to this phase of the Sumerian daily life is manual labor.

The records are far more complete for ancient India; except for the dance, and military training of nobility, however, their religious and philosophic teachings early sent these peoples along a path of rejection of vigorous bodily activity, although many other health teachings are found in religious instruction and in medical books written by the Hindu physicians. The only sports recorded were those engaged in by the military and the nobility, consisting of archery, fencing, and polo (a later addition which had its origins in India).

Sports were enjoyed by the typical Egyptian in ancient times, swimming being the most common to both sexes. Wrestling, charioteering, and gymnastics also were commonly pursued by the military class. Their sons received instruction in these and other activities at the barracks schools. Here as in the case of most of the ancient nations, sports were a part of religious ceremonies and practices. Hunting, although not considered as a sport in educational institutions became such, as tribal life merged into that of the nation. In *Before Philosophy* (2), the authors give a brief description of the early Egyptian: "The rooms are crammed and packed with vigorous scenes of life, and the lust for more life. The vizier is shown spearing fish, while his servants bring a bellowing hippopotamus to bay. (He) supervises the roping and butchering of cattle, the ploughing and harvesting of the fields, the carpenters and metal-workers in their shops, and the building of boats for his funeral services . . . he gives the impression of high potential, of being ready to spring into action . . . this is how he wants to be remembered; this is the good life he wishes to extend into eternity."

The *fifth* historical classification of physical activities dwells upon the Greeks. As in some other instances, the Greeks seem to burst upon the scene full blown, without the usual gradual development. But careful scholarship points to a debt to the Egyptians not only in art, architecture, a sense of geometric order and government organization, but also to the physically active life.

It seems reasonable to believe that the tap root of the Olympian Games, which included the physical activities reported by Homer in the ninth century B.C., (boxing, wrestling, weight-casting, spear throwing, running, chariot racing—all with religious connections), reaches back to tribal days when effectiveness in survival efforts included not only skill in weaponry but also hand-to-hand combat with an enemy or an animal. This particular development admits credibility when it is known that the spot on the Alpheus River, where the Olympian Games were later held, was sacred. It was the place where for years before the Games, religious ceremonies and athletic contests were held.

Confining consideration to Sparta and Athens, the children in both city states began their education at about the age of seven. Spartan children (girls and boys) of citizens were sent to state schools where they experienced ten years of preparation for military life. It consisted of wrestling, running, marching to music, discus and javelin throwing, swimming, hunting, rough games, choral and war dances. Forty years of soldiering were preceded by two years of scouting in which the individual survived by whatever means he could. All work in Sparta was performed by helots (slaves), with artistic, handcraft, commercial and intellectual activities being depreciated. Women were accepted on a par with men, being known throughout Greece for their strength, horsemanship and beauty in addition to their social position. The individual was valued as a military resource of the state.

In Athens, education was limited to sons of freemen and directed toward the "harmonious development of the whole man." Schools were private and parents decided on the amount of schooling their offspring should have. One of the three main emphases of the curriculum was

physical education which included posture training and a form of corrective physical education. At the age of eighteen the male youth became
an ephebe and was sent to the borders in garrison training, military
service and hunting. The boy began his instruction in physical education
at the palaestra or "wrestling school" where he learned to wrestle, box,
jump, run and engage in exercises under an instructor. The gymnasium
was also the site of discussions and exercise of adult men. Youths were
selected and trained for performance at festivals where, among other
activities, choral groups of young men participated—a distinctive honor.
It is clear that in comparison with the Spartan youth, the Athenian was no
match in physical activities. But, in terms of breadth of education the
Spartan could not be compared with the Athenian. On the other hand,
the Athenian male citizen spent most of his time at the gymnasium exercising and participating in verbal and social activities with other male
citizens. Engaging in many local athletic contests, in addition to preparing
for and participating in the three other national Games besides the Olympian, together with participating during the great many Athenian holidays, also helped insure the physical fitness of Athenian youth.

The *sixth* classification of physical activities when looked at historic-
ally, focuses on the Romans. Although it has been said, "Romans went
to school to the Greeks," they do not appear to have been apt students in
some respects. The early Romans were ambitious and warlike. Physical
training was a part of the education of every father's son, there being no
schools, yet beliefs were strong in the value of discipline, endurance,
strength, agility, hardihood and skill in such activities as horsemanship,
the javelin, shield, spear and sword. As may be apparent, this sort of
program resembles that of the Spartans, and of the Persians before them.
The early Romans never came to understand the Athenian idea of gymnastics for carriage, beauty, grace, symmetry and the harmonious development of the individual.

Even in their play, the sons of early Romans competed in boxing,
wrestling, jumping, running and swimming. Virgil is quoted as having
written, "We carry our children to the icy streams and harden them in
the bitter, icy water; as boys they spend wakeful nights over the chase, and
tire out the whirlwind. . . ." On reaching the age of seventeen, the Roman
youth was subject to military draft, serving until he was forty-seven if
needed and discharged when the war was over. During these years,
military games as exercise were severe and discipline was strict in such
activities as swimming-in-armor and naked, sham battles, horsemanship,
running, jumping and wrestling. For those who were not drafted, the
Campus Martius (a field outside the walls of the city) was used as a place

to practice sports, games and swimming. Because the Roman was a pragmatist, and, because physical activities which did not lead to some practical end were not understood, Romans never became skillful in activities such as running, dancing and boxing.

Although they left proud legacies of law, administration, engineering and architecture, the Roman legacy of physical activities-of-value was negative. Their influence on the Pan-Hellenic Games was negative, and they are usually regarded as responsible for the negative aspects of professionalism in sports. They accentuated brutality in the sports to the extent that the descriptive adjective "Roman" is still used to typify this aspect of sports.

The foregoing historical sketch suggests some implications at this time. As man made the effort to survive, three general factors or forces intermeshed. These were: the conditions and impact of the environment with which he reacted and which he used; his biological heritage; and, his proclivity to change some of that which he was, had, felt and thought. Man is, but he also is more than a product of his environment and his biological inheritance.

Mankind did many things. Not all of them dealt with reacting to and with the environment in accordance with his nature. He did some kinds of things that were different, ". . . acts of creation . . . to achieve some self-selected end . . ."(1) We shall use a practical illustration. He did not continue using only his bare hands or a chance-selected object as tools for fishing, fighting or fashioning a trap in hunting. Rather, he began to select objects that were suitable for the purpose at hand, or/and he created crude tools out of some material at hand. Later, he selected other materials that lasted longer or were more effective. He improved his tools by fashioning them in new, more efficient ways. New tools were invented to serve both new and old purposes. He tried new skills that increased the effectiveness of the tool-user. More suitable sites for tool manufacture were selected. Specializations developed that led to the division of labor. Esthetic decorations were made on tools to identify the symbols of the maker or in response to some "self-selected end," such as a particular design or a certain use of colored dyes.

As mankind performed workday and creative activities, he found it advantageous, a source of satisfaction and pleasurable to possess accuracy, steadiness, equilibrium, flexibility, skill, strength and endurance. It also seems reasonable to assume that he became at least somewhat aware of some of the observable characteristics of the highly-skilled performer in, for example, javelin-throwing as a sport or in warfare; in war or religious dances; or, in horsemanship. Today we use such terms as gracefulness, rhythmicality, beauty, efficiency, harmoniousness to indicate some of these characteristics that also became desired and wanted. Was not the last named characteristic elevated to the acme of prominence by the Athenian?

So wanted, desired, attractive, aspired for did these personal attainments become that they were among the most sought-after achievements in the culture. That is, they became among the highest *values* as value systems were gradually developed. And, except for the European "age of asceticism" and the impact of pessimism on some cultures of Eastern civilization, biological values accruing from sports, exercise and the dance are still prized possessions of even Technological man as typified by the American astronauts.

Nevertheless, mankind may have come to regard some or all biological outcomes of physical activity as values "in reverse." He first may have experienced consequences which were deleterious or fatal to the individual, family, tribe or nation because some individuals lacked physical fitness, abilities and capacities. The absence of these traits would be expected to bring dramatic reaction if their consequences consistently occurred and/or were highly traumatic. In fact, should he who was in possession of strength, endurance and other biological values lose, injure or lose control of some crucial body part (finger, hand, eye, foot, leg) how poignantly would such misfortune be felt by him and others affected by that kind of a loss or incapacity. The fact that the armies of such early "militaristic" nations as Sparta and Rome "retired" its soldiers as they reached an age when biological attributes were apt to be less dependable, speaks for the recognition of even possible losses as *disvalues*.

Thus, it may have been such negative conditions which helped to lead man to seek out the opposite conditions. Certainly, the combination of a desire to *avoid* the disvalues and a desire to *acquire* the values formed a force which catapulted biological values into prominence in the ways of life of developing man. It seems apparent that such values proved to be a recognized essential not only in war but also in such activities as religious dances, manual labor, festivals and in the schooling of the offspring of persons of affluence and position in emerging nations.

Thus, today, as many trustworthy relationships among mankind and between him and nature are still being sought, one of the most effective relationships in the fashioning of man has proven to be the emergence of biological values as a part of his life from at least Early Neolithic times down to national beginnings. The only early nation's history lacking hard evidence of the position occupied by sport, the dance and exercise in its culture, is Sumer. Sumerologists have translated only a fraction of the thousands of Sumerian clay tablets unearthed so far. As translations are extended, it seems reasonable to expect evidence that biological values were a part of that culture too.

## REFERENCES

1. Dubos, René. *Man Adapting*. New Haven, Conn.: Yale University Press, 1965, p. xviii.
2. Frankford, Henri et al. *Before Philosophy*. Chicago: University of Chicago Press, 1968, pp. 103–4.
3. Kramer, Samuel Noah. *History Begins at Sumer*. Garden City, N.Y.: Doubleday & Co., 1959, pp. 1–8.
4. Van Dalen, D. B., and Sasajima, Kohsuke. *Quest IV*, April 1965, pp. 68–77.

## READINGS

Augusta, Joseph and Burian, Zdenek. *Prehistoric Man*. London: Paul Hamign, 1960.

Berreman, Gerald et al. *Anthropology Today*. Del Mar, Calif.: CRM Books, 1971.

Coon, Carleton S. *The Story of Man*. New York: Alfred A. Knopf, 1955.

Ceram, C. W. *The March of Archaeology*. New York: Alfred A. Knopf, 1958.

Dubos, René. *So Human the Animal*. New York: Charles Scribner's Sons, 1968.

Fried, Morton H. *Readings in Anthropology*, vols. 1 and 2. New York: Thomas Y. Crowell Co., 1969.

Hackensmith, C. W. *History of Physical Education*. New York: Harper & Row Publishers, 1966.

Van Dalen, D. B. and Bennett, Bruce L. *A World History of Physical Education*. Englewood Cliffs, N. J.: Prentice-Hall, 1971.

# 4 | Physical Activity Values in the American Culture

WHAT IS the factor that is missing when it comes to explaining the dramatic differences between the physical activity programs of Athens and Sparta, in view of the general similarities in time, place, condition or circumstance? An answer is suggested later in this chapter.

In the previous chapter, again and again it was apparent that the physical activities of peoples together with attendant values were seen to change as times changed, as the general location changed, as conditions changed. An understandable response is, "Sure! Of course!" And, as this chapter proceeds, it will be observed that significant changes occur in periods varying greatly in length and distributed helter skelter. The gaps between these periods follow no neat pattern, no predictable spacing.

Also by way of introduction, although the concern of this book is with biological values, other values will be mentioned, man being indivisible. The value one selects for himself as he engages in sports, games, the dance and exercise are chosen from within the framework of the impacts made by all stimuli which act upon him. Man need not even be aware of them or have the ability to identify these values. Some of the stimuli come from the environment and carry titles like social, esthetic, political, psychological, economic or physical. Other stimuli that form the framework are internal, being based on his biological heritage. Psychological stimuli serve as a good example of the indivisibility of man as they also rest in part on biological heritage.

The third element in this framework from which man selects his values is what the human *does* with that which the other two "bring in." This third element also includes such things as the individual's potentialities, some of which neither he, she nor anyone else may be aware. Someone asked this question, "In the great days of ancient Rome, what Roman senator or man-of-the-mind would have pointed to an unknown Jew, in answer to a question, 'Who would change the world more than Caesar?' "

To know the biological values in American culture is far less important than also to *understand* them. But this latter suggests a consideration of at least the main forces and factors that led to these values. We would shortchange ourselves without the background of biological values related to the dance, exercise, and sports in American culture.

### BACKGROUND

From the close of the Roman Empire to the beginnings of the North American colonies is a leap of over a thousand years. One of the forces operating among the events of those times which had influence upon European peoples was their involvement in physical activities. There is a temptation to be content with that comment and to plunge immediately into the games, the dance, sports, exercise and manual labor of the colonists. But the European immigrants did not arrive bereft of traditions or lacking a background of beliefs about and experiences related to biological values.

The reader is warned that the next paragraphs make no pretence at comprehensiveness. Not only are they abbreviated but the time covered begins as recently as the Middle Ages. Later paragraphs cover the elapsed time from the Colonial period to the present day.

*European Beginnings.*   No neat chronology of the progress of physical activities and their values to Europeans, beginning with the Middle Ages, is feasible. The significant phenomenon is that most of the ideas, beliefs, proposals and value judgments about physical activities for the next 1,000 years after the Middle Ages are reflections of the teachings of such timeless giants as Hippocrates, Plato and Galen.

Starting with the feudalistic era, the knightly exercises or sports serve as an example of the physical activities of the time. A number of these activities antedate the Christian Era, springing from Homer's accounts of the funeral games, and, from the first Olympiads. The values related to these activities were rooted deeply in the beliefs and practices of Greeks lost in antiquity, according to C. W. Ceram (3). The knightly exercises carried on intermittently through the Reformation, the Renaissance, the

Enlightenment in Europe, thus preceding or paralleling the settling of the early colonists along the Atlantic western fringe of North America.

Useful ideas may disappear but they are not forever lost. Before Gutenberg's moving printing press and before hand-wrought messages were carved in stone, or tongue-to-ear legends, nonverbal gestures served as vehicles to carry man's evaluation of his experiences and his beliefs. And, wherever man walked the sands or sailed the seas, ideas and values also journeyed. Thus, the knightly exercises are found now and then, and, here and there, throughout many changing cultures, and with many differing values claimed for them.

*The Early Church's Views.*    There were arcs of time during which physical activities (except manual labor) all but vanished from the Western world. One such era is identified by some as the Age of Asceticism, when the Church "subjugated the flesh," as Rome's social institutions disintegrated. Some accounts of this period have been presented in harsh terms. Modern scholarship suggests a more controlled view. For example, Ralph B. Ballou, Jr. (2), asked fifty-six carefully selected modern scholars to examine the writings of fifty "pre-eminent authors" of the early Church. His chief finding was that in spite of some cases of extreme asceticism in some monasteries, the reflected basic attitude was that the good or ill of physical activity depended on the way it was used. He also found that in monasteries in which these extreme instances occurred, other local Church brothers were in opposition to such measures.

There were, however, strong Western church leaders who opposed sports, the dance, exercise and games, and the values claimed for them. They opposed such activities in the Church schools' curricula, except for lay students. In the meantime, in pagan schools such activities were provided for the students, and, early Western churchmen who had been educated in the Eastern Empire, also favored them. The substance of this period therefore is that it was a time when physical activities were seldom seen in Church schools. It was a time when the devout spent and were encouraged to spend much time in spiritual, spiritually-oriented and spiritually-intended activities. (The Church fathers understandably remembered the consequences of the Roman excesses of a *"physical"* nature.) At the same time, it must be considered as significant that *exceptions* to the Church's restraints kept alive Western man's desire to express himself, using the avenues of expression for mental, economic, political, social, and physical activities. These were soil and seed and root for the Renaissance.

*Eminent "Spokesmen" and Their Proposals.*    As the media of civilization were gradually restored in the West, almost without exception, doctors of medicine, essayists, educationalists, artists, noblemen, church-men, and reformers advocated participation in programs of physical activities. They saw in such involvement desirable outcomes (values) to the individual and to the social order.

Thanks to Arabian scholars, translations of Aristotle and Plato were made, and later became available to Catholic monks who in turn translated these papers into Latin. Thus, engaging in muscular activity had a respectable base for the views and the reasons of the "Spokesmen." In addition, the knightly sports filled the need for an example of a program which had proved to be effective. The third support for this rather astonishing group of reformers, instigators and backers of sports, the dance, and exercise was the word of Galen, Marcus Aurelius' personal physician, who wrote at length on the values of muscular activity in the second century A.D.

Who were some of these men who laid the foundation for Europe's awakening to and reviving of the importance of such activities? To merely mention their names emphasizes the unusual fact that for these centuries men, who knew virtually nothing, technically, about physical education, athletics and the dance, promoted and supported them. They also stimulated participation in, as well as public backing and approval of this matrix of today's programs of athletics, recreation and physical education. Here is a partial listing of these men (without concern for chronology): Hieronymous Mercurialis, King Richard III of England, Pope Pius II, Ignatius de Loyala, King Henry VIII of England, John Calvin, Martin Luther, Comenius, Roger Asham, Montaigne, Rabelais, Rousseau, Thomas Elyot, Locke, da Feltre, Pestalozzi, Basedow, la Giocosa, Mulcaster, Vergerius, Erasmus and Juan Luis Vives. Such an array should not be used as a basis for concluding that all men of the intellect of the times agreed with them. We do not know. But the directions charted by these men reactivated a journey begun by the Greeks a millennium before. Here we have the answer to the question asked in this chapter's initial paragraph. In addition to time, place and condition, the missing factor in explaining cultural changes and differences is *human beings with ideas, possessed of courage and capable of dynamic action.*

Following the above pattern of briefly synthesizing main points, what sorts of physical activities did these personages, *collectively,* favor, support, write about, or initiate? Here is not only the activity-heritage of the Europeans emigrating to America but also what was to become the exercise, sports, games and dance program in the U.S.A. What were some of the European elements of these programs and their values, beginning roughly with the Middle Ages? The knightly sports which spawned military and social values through dancing, tennis, quoits, crossbow, ball games, swimming, rope and ladder climbing, wrestling, running, spear-throwing, archery, battle axe, mace, broadsword, lance and shield, horsemanship (including that in full armor), jousting and tournaments. Peasants joined the noblemen and the trainees in hunting and falconry, high and broad jumping, and actual warfare. The peasant's usual physical activity was manual labor although some became so skillful in making and repairing armor of metal and leather, and other offensive and defensive equipment, that they became specialists in this sort of skilled labor. The other exception was the wandering entertainers—acrobats, tumblers, dancers, jugglers and tight-rope walkers.

As the merchant class and guilds developed, enjoying greater freedom and self-determination, feudalism declined and towns grew in number and population. Among the desires of the people was an education for their children. Although "practical" schools were developed for the guildsman's children, religious, social and intellectual emphases were not forgotten. However, there was no place in the curricula for games, sports, exercise or dance. These activities developed *outside* the school and became a part of the life of the people, and a part of their leisure time—in addition to aiding military preparedness. Contests were held between guildsmen from nearby towns—the beginning of athletic competition between "town teams" and eventually the professional leagues in various sports so common today in the U.S.A. Some of the sports were so rough they were declared illegal. Some of these are included in the list of activities which typified the times: football, archery, running games, wrestling, ice-skating, foot races, the beginning of rugby, "casting the stone", battle royal fist-fighting, bowling, ball games, handball, and forerunners of golf and cricket.

In contrast to the well-defined values of the knightly sports, no such specificity of values accompanied the physical activity programs during the post-feudal period. Primarily, they served as a release, entertainment, catharsis and a diversion. They also were used by the Church for morale building and for unifying purposes. And, through participation in these activities, some peasants and guildsmen hoped to attain religious, social and recreational outcomes (values) and to achieve the still-important military value as well.

*Changes Come* (6).    As the early universities in Europe emerged from the monastic and church schools, no provision for physical education was made. Nor did the university authorities encourage participation in them as extra-curricular pursuits. But the period of scholasticism was not left without resources for keeping alive student participation in physical activities. Students from all over Europe were attracted to the universities, each bringing his locality's typical games, sports and the dance, in defiance of the authorities. That such student activities were not made a part of the curriculum at the time is not surprising.

Nevertheless, in Italy, the seat of a number of the first universities, the ferment and lure of freedom of thought, augmented by "different" ideas and "new" kinds of values brought in by the immigrating students, plus the "new" acquaintanceship with Greek and Roman classics, ushered in individual humanistic theories of education by the fifteenth and sixteenth centuries. As this movement crept northward, the "individual" emphasis lost its force within a short century as it met the influence of a deep concern for the welfare of others in the northern states. Thus, social humanism became the chief theory of education throughout most of Europe. This was not the first time that individual freedom, self-expression and emphasis by the individual on himself proved an inadequate and unsuccessful guide in education or in a way of life, as Frankfort et al (5) reveals. The idea was two thousand years old. It failed then also.

What views and proposals were made by humanists about physical activities in European education? There was a revival of interest in the knightly sports. These formed a loose foundation for the proposals of most of the humanists, some of whose names appear on page 39. In addition, there were such proposals as the following for noblemen's sons: military-like exercises for very young boys in anticipation of later wars but gearing the amount and severity to the boy's age up to puberty. The daily time allotment for boys engaging in physical activities varied from thirty minutes daily to three hours, adapted to age level. Some advocated that academic work and the exercise-sports program be interspersed. Others thought that the activity program should be nonfatiguing for the student. There was some opposition to dancing for boys, while other humanists objected to any exercises for military preparedness. Long, rapid walks and mountain-climbing were two activities suggested for the children's program. A suggestion was made that a program inducing relaxation was needed. Activities for educational purposes, introduction of concern for the safety of participants, and exercises for handicapped children were other proposals, anticipating Pehr H. Ling. One humanist advocated that children be given the exercises which their parents engaged in so that the former would be more skilled by the time they reached adulthood.

Some humanists proposed compulsory participation in activities while others took the contrary view. One proposal made in the sixteenth century was that children be classified for engaging in outdoor games and

sports and exercises. There were varied suggestions as to the programs'
emphases, such as "nimbleness," "elasticity," "full development of the
limbs," "sense of joy," "strong, healthy men-of-action," "personal fitness," "a sound mind in a sound body" (borrowing from Juvenal), individual activities that developed "social benefits," and "development of the
five senses" as tools of the intellect. A proposal was also made to the
effect that physical play be supervised. One well-known humanist suggested that the education of children consist of nothing but physical
activities for the first twelve years of life. One *avant garde* idea was that
"proper health habits" be inculcated in the physical education program
(borrowing from Comenius).

   *Biological Values of the Eminent "Spokesmen."* A gross summary
of the major values implied or acknowledged, directly or indirectly, by
the eminent European "Spokesmen" listed on page 39, from twelfth-
century feudalism through the years paralleling the colonial period in
America, include the following: for the persons of the lowest economic
class in feudal times whose chief physical activity was manual labor, the
major values were survival and occasional diversion. Through their work
they also helped their masters "survive" at the economic level to which
they were accustomed. Later, the merchant class, and, after the start of
the Industrial Revolution, the industrialists were similarly helped to "survive." A related value of the peasants and serfs was assisting their masters
in military forays and defenses or preparing for such. The chief values
of physical activity for the knights and noblemen in addition to military
readiness and chivalry, were the development of courage, stamina and
religion-related values. Chivalry, as recognized today, served as a step
in the direction of a more civilized people. One of the values that gradually re-emerged at this time was "health." This Hippocrates-Plato-Galen-
anticipated value of physical activities was all but overlooked for a thousand years until these postfeudal times. At about the same time, "physical
welfare of the individual," "hygiene," "physical well-being," "proper
habits of health," and a dozen similar ideas were proposed by some of the
"Spokesmen."

   At the time, a good many of these leaders regarded "the self-improve-
ment of the individual" as a prime value. Later, "social relationships"
was recognized as a value as such statments as: "children playing together," "brotherly feelings," and "social competence" were made. There
also was a period reminiscent of ancient Greece, when high-level skills
were regarded as a most worthy attainment and thus represented a major
value to those who sensed it. Some other values recognized by the Europeans of these times form a loose cluster of values. They are: "endurance,"

"hardihood," "muscle toughness," "harden against weather changes," "personal fitness," "fitness to perform," "strength," "vigorous body" and "physical development."

The relationship of the physical to the other aspects of man, i.e., the "whole man concept," is another value of participation in physical activities pointed out by some of the European "Spokesmen." Here are some additional statements which reveal at least implied values which they saw in such participation: "harmonious bodily development"; "education should include all phases of man including the physical"; "include bodily exercise with mental and moral training"; "character training through physical activities"; "perform skillfully all of life's activities"; "don't fashion the soul without fashioning the body"; "usefullness of exercises for both mind and body"; "the body is the tabernacle of the mind"; "limbs, the senses and bodily organs should be exercised"; "moral and physical development should be simultaneous"; "the program of activities is pleasurable"; "both body and soul have been created by the hand of God"; "give equal emphasis to the moral influence of physical activities"; "exercise helps train the whole being and for preparing the individual for his role as a citizen"; "participation in physical activities is as important as daily mental activities"; "education develops all the main faculties including the physical"; "educate the physical at the same time as his mind"; " 'tis not a body that we are training up, but a man"; "train the mind only insofar as the body permits"; "develop health and strength of body, integrity, sense-acuity and self-responsibility as tools of the mind"; "mental vigor is aided by physical vigor"; and, "put equal stress on the mental, moral and physical."

*European Specialists in Physical Education.* The focal force of the ideas and proposals of the "Spokesmen" found targets not only in European schools, universities and the life-styles of the people, but also on European men who were or became specialists in physical education as a career(9). Toward the close of the eighteenth century and a good deal of the nineteenth these men made themselves increasingly heard. Individually, each of them made worthy and distinctive contributions to and valuable modifications in this field. Collectively, they and their immediate representatives gave impetus to the concepts, practices and values of physical education in the United States. As we shall see, the peak of this thrust was reached in this country fifty years after it had been reached in Europe.

In the long look, the Specialists appeared on the scene at generally the same period. Some of the names and nationalities may be of passing interest at least: *Germany:* Johann Friedrich Guts Muths, Gerhard Vieth, Friedrich Ludwig Jahn, Friedrich Froebel, Adolph Spiess, Emil Harwick; *Sweden:* Pehr Henrik Ling, Lars Gabriel Branting, Hjalmar Ling; *Denmark:* Franz Nachtegall; *Switzerland:* Philipp Emanuel von Fellenberg, Jacques Dalcroze; *France:* Clement Joseph Tissot, Francois Delsarte; *Great Britain:* Archibald Maclaren.

*European Specialists' Proposals.* What sorts of ideas and programs did these specialists propose? For the most part their proposals came during a period of acute nationalistic awareness among the peoples of their respective countries. It is not astonishing that *systems* of physical education grew out of this kind of concern. All of these men knew (or could have known) of the views of the "Spokesmen" who preceded or were contemporary with them, as well as the contributions of others as far back as the ancient Greeks. The influence of the educational reformers and theorists of the times catapulted the thinking of most of these Specialists in novel directions. In some instances, the politico-geographic positions of their countries directed their efforts to shaping their proposals in accord with military values. Most of these men were strong leaders, had great zeal and enthusiasm, and an acute dedication and unshakable confidence in their ideas and their respective causes. Such factors also accentuated their tendency to develop *systems* rather than general plans for programs of physical education. These same factors led to some spirited differences between and among these men and their followers.

Again, acknowledging the lack of an orderly chronology of these proposals, here are some of the physical activities and ideas about them which came from the pens, voices and actions of the Specialists, collectively: creative exercises; prescribed exercises on apparatus and with equipment such as horizontal bars, chest weights, balance beam, high bar, wooden horse, climbing ropes, ladders and poles, rope ladders, stall bars, moving beam, wand, boom, vaulting buck, jumping-vaulting pole, standards, pits, dumbbells, Indian clubs, light and heavy weights, inclined rope, Swedish horizontal bar; and natural equipment such as trees and fences. All of the systems using such equipment also included at least a few games, sports, and the dance. The British program consisted almost entirely of games and sports. The other countries turned to this source when their specialists felt the need for the social values. In like fashion, when Great Britain felt the need to increase the physical condition of its military forces, it turned to one or another of the three systems (German, Danish or Swedish). Some of the physical activities of a sports type of this era were: baseball-like games, fencing, swimming, soccer, horseback-riding, cricket, bowling, hunting, skating, skiing, track and field, polo, rugby, hockey, quoits, golf, fishing, tennis, falconry, rowing, wrestling and boxing. The dance and eurythmics also were popular. The Swedish corrective-medical gymnastics program initiated by Pehr H. Ling brought still a different and important aspect of physical activity as well as unique values.

Some of the significant results of the work of the Specialists and their representatives became possible through their use of some of the teaching methodology of the "new" education which roughly paralleled the beginning and continuation of European physical education of that period. It was this "new" education, in fact, which placed so much value upon physical education that it was made a part of the curriculum in most schools as well as a distinctive part of the lives of the peoples of most European nations.

*Biological Values as Seen by the European Specialists.* Without regard to comparative claims of the Specialists for the values of their respective systems or specific physical activities, what, collectively, were these values? The two values most consistently highlighted were "health" and the "physical improvement" of the individual. Physical education's "contribution to his aggregate education" was another value frequently acknowledged. "Different kinds of physical attainments gained from regular participation" was still another (not wholly unexpected) acknowledged value. As at other times and places, it was regarded as especially worthwhile for the individual to possess such attributes as physical skills, strength, endurance, dexterity, flexibility, and the like. One of the more important values was that outcomes such as these attributes helped to "restore and/or preserve nationhood," and, to "anticipate threats from other nations." But even the peoples of weaker, smaller nations came to believe that games and sports contributed to fostering "freedom of choice," "freedom of expression," the "democratic way and democratic ideals."

A cluster of sociopsychological values also were recognized as being related to participation in athletics, the dance, and physical education. Here are some of these other values: esthetic, political, social-moral and educational. Even the public of these times and places put value upon such subvalues as: "beauty"; "gracefulness"; "movement responses to music"; "discipline and self-discipline"; "social competence"; "self-reliance"; "initiative"; "self-confidence"; "valor"; "patriotism"; "sense of responsibility"; "freedom"; "group unity"; "cooperation"; "adapting activities to the individual's condition and age"; "fair competition"; "adjusting the program to handicapped children"; "correcting remediable defects"; "arranging activities from easy to difficult"; "character development"; "enjoyment"; "leadership-followership"; "activities in the outdoors"; "senses-development"; "activities that carried over to leisure time"; and "sportsmanship."

The European systems and programs of physical activities led to the formation of clubs, societies, organized groups. Some of these were interested in but one activity, such as rowing, for example. Others of these organizations were interested in an entire system or an entire program such as gymnastics. To this day one organization continues to promote Ling's corrective-medical program, with a worldwide meeting held once every decade, called "the Lingiad." Such organizations with their fostering of socialization is an example of a ready-made product being transplanted to the United States somewhat later, and serving as a social force in the twentieth century. The German Turnverein is another example of an organization's promoting a social value in which the participating members believed.

### PHYSICAL ACTIVITIES AND BIOLOGICAL VALUES OF AMERICAN COLONISTS

The first English settlers in 1607* along the western edge of the Atlantic Ocean, were a heterogeneous lot, economically, educationally, religiously, politically, and culturally. That there should have been major difficulties within and among these colonies before, during and after the Revolutionary War is understood without difficulty. One of the few things these first immigrants had in common was their lack of knowledge, skills and know-how for survival. They brought with them such insufficient amounts of food that many suffered famine. The soil in some of the colonies was very poor, with scanty harvests as a consequence. Diseases became epidemic. Personal clothing often was inadequate. Frequently dwellings were poorly constructed and inadequate in number, size and protection.

Some colonists proved to be uncooperative, refusing to share and help in the common safety, welfare and livelihood. Leaders had to enforce work orders by meting out severe punishments. In some New England colonies the Puritan church strongly opposed idleness and wantonness. Strong measures were used to stamp out amusements, entertainment and pleasures. Other colonists began to grow weary of the long hours of hard work without diversions and also became recalcitrant. In spite of

---

* Raleigh and Gilbert in 1578–87 made unsuccessful voyages to establish English Colonies in North America.

increasingly severe punishments, some men continued to break the laws against wantonness and idleness. Some tradesmen forsook their stores on occasion even in the face of being condemned to the galleys. Nevertheless, a few of the colonies began to be more strongly organized and established. In such cases, the laws were softened. Jamestown, Virginia was such a colony. In New England, the reverse was the case. The church and the court became aware that as more colonists arrived, the greater became the opposition to the restrictive laws. All phases of the lives of the settlers from the Massachusetts Bay and Connecticut colonies were placed under the scrutiny and judgment of church and court. But not all such measures accomplished their purpose. For example, the church began to require attendance on Thursday evenings, providing more opportunities for prayer, worship, and "visiting." However, numbers of the men were soon doing their visiting at taverns.

*Physical Activities of Early Colonists.* But such an account of early life in some of the colonies omits those physical activities which had biological values, even though perhaps not recognized as such by the colonists. Except on the Sabbath, walking in the fields or on the street was permitted in the restrictively governed colonies. On the occasional holidays some settlers engaged in dancing, wrestling, foot-races and contests of physical prowess. England's King James II in 1618, in disagreement with the Puritans in England, approved of dancing, archery, leaping, vaulting, May games, Morris dances, ball games, and "other sports." Bowling, and bull-and-bear-baiting were barred. The Puritans in England who opposed games, sports and dancing received no support from Calvin, a bowling enthusiast. John Milton consistently supported "the joyous aspects of life." Some of the Puritans in England expressed disagreement with the restrictions placed on life activities by colonial Puritans, to no avail.

One factor that a brief account of the New England Puritan colonies may overlook is indicated by the historical view to the effect that the strict laws and sternly enforced customs helped immeasurably in the survival of the early English colonies. Eventually, however, the English proclivity for sports and the dance became activated and so was instrumental in determining the life-style of most of the English colonists. The early Dutch and French colonies were not plagued by restrictive laws, and from the beginning enjoyed the games, sports and dances of their native countries.

*Physical Activities of Eighteenth-Century Colonists.* By the start of the eighteenth century, a century after the beginnings of English colonization, the pastimes, games, sports and dances among the new Americans provided a picture of a lusty, vigorous, extroverted, independent yet neighborly, hard-working people. Some of the following physical activities are recreational more than they are productive of biological values. Nevertheless, these, together with the strictly physical activities, aid in understanding the later colonist who synthesized his work, worship, war-related and recreational activities into a way of life.

Here then are some of these activities of the later colonists(4): fencing, buggy- and sleigh-riding, wrestling, horse-racing, shooting, country dancing, hunting, gauff (golf), boating and boat-racing, shuttle-cocks, target practice (with guns), handball, cricket, horse-man racing, bowling-on-the-green, horse racing, log rolling, sledding, wagon shows, barn-raising, Morris dancing, ball playing, country fairs, fishing, social and sports clubs, husking bees, football, nine pins, swimming, tennis, shuffle-board, foot races, boxing, house-raising, skating and racing, cock-fighting, dancing schools, hockey, greased pig chasing, ice carnivals, circuses, cudgeling, beauty contests, musical contests, whist, magic lantern showing, serenades, oratorical contests, acrobatics, barefoot fighting, billiards, holiday festivals, plays, dice-rolling, and backgammon.

*Some Major Values.* This listing of physical activities and leisure-time diversions and entertainments, incomplete though it is, suggests that during the seventeenth and eighteenth centuries the focus of the colonists' physical activity had shifted from the area of survival value to that of a combination of the development and maintenance of the welfare of the individual, and the beginnings of the socialization and acculturation of the people.

With the appearance of some of the same games, sports and dances that were first engaged in within European nations and the shift in the colonists' major values just mentioned, the impact of European life upon colonial life is readily apparent. It also seems reasonable to assume that this transfer did not stop with only these kinds of activities. European beliefs and some features in life-styles, as well as social institutions such as education (though not all of them) were also carried over from their original native shores. Additionally, in the new environment, the various kinds and nationalities of European peoples with novel problems to meet and solve—the meeting of peoples from other native lands with their "strange" ways, beliefs and values, and, never forgetting the confirmed purposes of coming to a new land—all coalesced into the making of *Americans.* One aspect of this coalescing of ideas, ideals, life-styles and aspirations was, of course, the adoption and absorption of the physical activities and teaching methods which had been developing in Europe. Into this complexity of influences, it also must be remembered, were the

Renaissance, the Church, the Reformation, the Naturalistic and guild schools, the "Spokesmen" and the Specialists. The printed page, the flow of immigrants, and the return to Europe of an occasional colonial personage who upon his return to the colonies brought back "the new," combined to form a surge and continuance of change, to a people already "busy with all their hands" trying to adapt to and fashion a stable nation of their own.

By the latter part of the eighteenth century, American grammar schools and academies were being founded. Both types of schools favored programs of physical education—after school hours. Some activities offered were: swimming, shinny, skating, ball games. The avowed values were: health and proper physical growth.

### NINETEENTH CENTURY AMERICAN PHYSICAL ACTIVITIES AND BIOLOGICAL VALUES

*Pre–Civil War Physical Activities and Values.** As the nineteenth century began, the citizenry of the budding nation was participating generally in physical activities similar to those of the Pre–Revolutionary War colonists, in contrast to the program found in the academies. These latter tended to follow the European influences even to the construction of gymnastic apparatus and outdoor gymnasiums, and pointed to the benefits in terms of military value as the outcome of their gymnastic programs.

Paralleling that part of the academy movement which included physical education in the curriculum were successful efforts to start educational institutions for women—referred to at the time as seminaries. Among the first of these were three that included physical education in their curricula. The three women responsible for this accomplishment were Emma Willard, Mary Lyon and Catharine Beecher. Collectively, dancing, exercises and calisthenics were introduced into women's education by these three early innovators. The values attached to their programs were "health," and "graceful, poised body dynamics." Oberlin College at about this time initiated calisthenics for women.

Another noteworthy event marks this era; namely the hiring of trained male instructors for the first time, as well as the use of some skilled gymnasts from Germany who had worked with Jahn. Within a few years several American universities and preparatory schools for boys adopted the German System, adding to it such sports as boxing, running, hiking, and fencing. The "gymnastic fad" collapsed but was revived two decades

---

* See Reference titles 7 and 8.

later through the public support of men like Jefferson, Franklin, and Horace Mann who not only pointed out the health and physical development values of this form of physical activity, badly needed by young men and boys, but also indicated that this exercise program should be made a part of the education of youth. In addition, about this time, school boys became interested in athletic sports, and in those cities with a goodly proportion of Germans, the German System of gymnastics was well established.

However, aside from these few exceptions, the first half of the nineteenth century and up to the Civil War is known as a rather slack period for participation in outdoor games and sports by American citizenry. This despite the invention of baseball, the publication of a number of books on exercises (two of which were written by Catharine Beecher and by Dio Lewis), the founding of the Y.M.C.A., the support of Herbert Spencer, and the spread of games and sports programs to additional universities. The values of the times were: health, the development of physical adequacy, social relationships, diversion, catharsis, and the educational value of physical education.

What force or forces could have contravened such an array of values and support of physical education and athletics? At least six events or conditions appear to have been responsible. Let us briefly recognize them.

1. Workers were drained from the rural areas to the cities, as these men sought the hard cash of possible employment in industry and business. The cities were totally unprepared to provide facilities, equipment, programs, or opportunity for participation not only in the physical activities familiar to these men, but in any other physical activities. During after-work hours and many and long periods of unemployment, there was nothing for these men to do.

2. Hordes of immigrants were arriving at accelerated rates, also drawn to the cities by possible employment. Except in "German" cities, there were also no provisions for the immigrants to engage in the physical activities of their native lands and nothing resembling an American program of games, sports, or exercise.

3. Civic leadership, at the time, did not even recognize the existence of a problem.

4. The growing recognition of the values of physical activities by colleges and schools made little or no impact upon those in civic leadership positions.

5. Commercially-minded men saw, recognized, and grasped the opportunity to offer amusements and entertainment, paid for by the "customer." Dance halls were built. Entertainment of many kinds were made

available for "watchers." Opportunities quickly developed where gambling on anything from a horse race to a cock-fight appeared at every hand.

6. Men of questionable purpose and character associated themselves with such enterprises, including commercialized sports. This situation brought about two unfortunate results. Men possessed of athletic ability and devotees of exercise began to be held in low esteem by "decent folks." America began to become a nation of spectators. The exception was the wealthy class, and even the physical activities of that group were predominantly of the "sitting" type. It was not stylish to engage in exercise of active sports, though dancing was popular.

*Post–Civil War Changes.* The decades following the Civil War were in contrast to those preceding it to the extent that participation in physical activities was concerned. A veritable upsurge in interest and involvement in games, sports and the dance occurred as they acquired attendant values. Sports clubs sprang up promoting certain sports such as golf and tennis in every city, with men of the economy's middle-class as well as the wealthy industrialists and merchants, as members. It also became stylish for everybody to play, bicycle and row. The middle-class wanted to, had some of the leisure time for, and could now afford to do what the upper class did. Suddenly, to be a mere spectator was not enough. The increased participation which resulted helped eradicate some socioeconomic class prejudices. A widening in interest and support of cultural and educational enterprises followed. People began to learn that participation in physical activities not only elicited biological values, but also that one great value—enjoyment, once some skill and other requisites were acquired. Sports that everybody could play became popular. The democratic way took on new meanings for the typical citizen. Roller-skating swept the country along with croquet. Co-educational and outdoor activities also appealed to young and old, men and women, upper- and middle-class alike.

Also in contrast to the first half of the nineteenth century, colleges and universities began to influence the citizenry to engage in this program of activities. Part of this came from the invention of volleyball and basketball at the YMCA College at Springfield, Massachusetts. College football became a popular spectator sport even though college administrations remained unenthusiastic about intercollegiate athletic competition.

Part of sports' expansion during this period was due to the return of military servicemen who had become acquainted with and developed skills in some sports in nonactive days behind the lines. In addition, civic leaders by this time began to assume some responsibility for providing support for facilities and opportunities to sustain healthful outdoor activities. These leaders also joined some of the wealthy class in the removal of some of the social barriers by means of sports participation. Again, the YMCA was a leader in promoting sports and popular exercise programs. Still another favorable factor was the arrival in this country of skilled advocates of Swedish medical gymnastics which were readily accepted and adopted, particularly in New England, along with the Swedish light gymnastics.

The Swedish system attempted to provide a scientific approach to physical education, and for this reason a feeling of respect was associated with it. The Swedish emphasis upon giving physical examinations to school children, a new "first" for the United States, helped develop a favorable public image for the Swedish system.

Soon after the Civil War the YMCA officially added a "physical improvement" feature to its overall program, consisting of a balance between German and Swedish gymnastics, coupled with an attempt to make the program as attractive as possible. Under the leadership of Luther Halsey Gulick, two decades later, emphasis was placed upon sports, leading not only to the invention of basketball and volleyball, but also the formation of the Athletic League of North America. But, in spite of the expansion in sports' participation and interest, by the time of the first Modern Olympian Games in 1896, the United States fielded no official team. Nevertheless, sufficient numbers of United States men in track and field volunteered, many paying their own expenses, and swept that part of the Games.

Further evidence of the growing interest in sports, exercise and the dance during the latter part of the nineteenth century was the effort and support provided by communities and leaders of German extraction to motivate state legislatures to pass laws requiring physical education in schools. Although this venture was but partially successful, attention was called to comparative values between the German and Swedish systems. This led to some professional feuding, with some American physical educators taking sides, as the public schools, colleges and universities included programs of physical education in their offerings. However, W. G. Anderson, M.D., called the meeting in 1885 from which the American Association for the Advancement of Physical Education was formed. Through the stature (and tact) of Dudley A. Sargent, M.D., the "systems" feud did not lead to a dissolving of the new Association.

Sargent had become a respected leader in physical education areas before that episode, having developed a series of body measurements together with mechanical devices for testing and measuring muscular strength. He also initiated a voluntary program of physical education at Harvard for individuals, based on the student's showing on the tests used, along with anthropometric measurements required of all freshmen. These tests and measurements were valid enough to be used to help select athletes for Harvard varsity athletic squads. The devices employed have served researchers occasionally up to the present time.

The increase in numbers who participated in sports led to a new type of spectator, the man who could perform creditably in at least one sport and who watched athletes in other sports, with an appreciation and understanding of their skills, biological values, and other needed requisites.

In the 1880s and 1890s indoor and outdoor facilities sprang up in numbers sufficient to meet the great need for them. Bleachers, indoor tracks, showers, bowling alleys sprang up not only on college campuses, but also in public places, for public use. Again—the college administrations continued to withhold support for athletic programs on many campuses, particularly for football. In the meantime, however, ice hockey, basketball, swimming, cricket, English rugby, tennis, golf and lacrosse were added to college athletic programs.

One reason college administrations opposed varsity athletics was because they lacked control—over sports events, the eligibility of players, and the conduct of sports fans and sometimes of the athletes themselves. This condition led to the beginning of the formation of organizations whose function was to exercise control over such matters. For example, the Athletic League of North America, referred to above, continued to exert its good influence, the AAU was organized to attempt to supervise a number of sports, as was the ICAAAA for track and field sports' supervision.

Still another index of the extended participation in exercise, the dance and sports was the great lack of professionally trained men and women to fill the need for instructors in and administrators of these programs. Dio Lewis' Normal Institute was the first teacher-preparation venture, followed shortly by the Gymnastic Union Normal, the YMCA's International Training School and others.

In the fourth century B.C., at his health center on the Greek Isle of Cos, Hippocrates, the Father of Medicine, practiced the belief that physical activities were more healthful when performed outdoors. The idea has persisted. It is understandable that towns and cities in the United States began to use their plazas, greens, squares and fairgrounds as gathering places for outdoor physical activities, such as had been done in European towns and cities. By the close of the nineteenth century, the Playground Movement in the United States was, unofficially, well under way. By then, civic leaders had come to believe that the welfare of individuals and society was served if children had chances to play. Physicians and other careful observers publically took the position that the growth and development of children was favorably related to play. The evils of child labor began to be attacked. The stage was set not only for civic provisions for playgrounds, but also for corrective physical education. Churches, the YMCA and the YWCA, settlement houses, Turner societies, and socially-minded citizens and organizations began promoting not only municipal recreation, but also what today is called outdoor education, including camping, summer camps, state and federal parks.

Two further examples of the amplification of participation in physical activities in the latter part of the nineteenth century illustrates the degree to which this program was being developed. First were the provisions for these programs made by churches. Free exercise classes, basketball, social dancing and bowling are examples of some of the activities which were part of their programs. Some churches added gymnasiums and others converted or rented space in order that these activities might be made available. The other example is the to-be-expected accelerated involvement in the dance, as well as exercise and sports by and for women. Reference has been made to these programs in colleges, universities and the early seminaries, but noneducationally connected physical activity programs also became popular. Bicycling, bowling, basketball, track and field, hiking, mountain climbing, archery and golf are examples of activities which proved to be popular with the women. The beginnings of American dance and the continuation of folk dances from "the old country" also were enjoyed. This movement was but one indication of new ventures being undertaken by the women of the times in expressing individual freedom and a concern for their welfare.

*Post–Civil War Biological and Other Values of Physical Activities.* Such values as health, physical development and "sound bodies" in the latter half of the nineteenth century continued to be emphasized but now the responsibility for the emergence of these values was placed more and more on the doorsteps of educational institutions. In fact, so important did these values become that they were considered worthy of attention by the state and federal governments. Part of this overall emphasis came from physicians and physiologists. The value of play for children was highlighted by pediatricians and psychologists, as well as by some educators. There seemed to be the general agreement among these experts that play was related positively to normal growth and development of children. This also was the period when recognition began to be given the value of supervised physical activities for the correction of remediable defects, poise and carriage, and the contributory benefits of such activities to the mental health and rehabilitation of persons with certain pathological conditions.

The place of physical skills as helpful in enabling persons to prevent accidents also began to be noticed. Another matter of observation was that participation in sports aided in helping immigrants and those from rural areas adjust to city life when facilities, opportunities and leadership was provided. This bringing together of peoples not only contributed to social intercourse but also to helping peoples gain a better sense of citizenship in a developing democracy. And, the emphasis on outdoor spaces for children and adults to relax or play was regarded by physicians as a health asset.

## PHYSICAL ACTIVITIES AND ATTENDANT VALUES* IN TWENTIETH-CENTURY AMERICA

*An Extension of Values of Physical Activity.* From time to time throughout the previous pages values other than the biological have been mentioned. As the population increased, as school laws required children and youth to remain in attendance for more years, as the Morrill Act increased the number of public colleges at tuition rates and curriculums attractive to more students, and as the professional preparation of physical education instructors improved, many more young persons were enabled to experience for longer periods the values of participating in physical activities. Paralleling this development was the improvement in kinds and amounts of knowledge about man as a biological, as well as a social and psychological animal. Among those who recognized the worth of the inherent values of man's physical aspects, as well as other values besides the biological, were such personages as C. S. Peirce, G. S. Hall, W. L. Wundt, Will James, C. H. Judd and E. L. Thorndike. John Dewey, first as an educator and later as a philosopher, also opened doors for physical educationalists to see the social and sociological implications inherent in their work. The work of these personages revealed and led to some of the same sorts of values that were conjectures of the "Spokesmen" of more than a century before, such as the health, growth and development—mentally and socially—of children and youth. But, these twentieth-century "Spokesmen" had the advantage of possessing more hard, supportive evidence. So, once again, the wholeness of man, the interdependence and intermingling and the inseparability of the "parts"

---

* See Reference title 10.

of man and society were recognized, accepted and applied by physiologists, sociologists, psychologists and somewhat later, by physical educators.

*Some Disvalues.* As the spread and intensification of sports participation continued, highly skilled athletes attended college after years of high and preparatory school athletic competition, or began to be attracted to professional teams. Paralleling this development was an increase in the number of high school and college athletic conferences activated in part by an attempt to control or eliminate some of the malpractices which began to threaten amateurism in American school and college sports. Though high school and college administrators and some others became concerned over such conditions, the citizenry in general seemed little concerned. The practice of showing one's loyalty to a college or professional team by attending its athletic events became commonplace. Thus, America began again to suffer from "spectatoritis." As desirable as it appeared, to attend the sports events of one's college, high school or professional team, the result in recent years has been that scores of millions of Americans watch these contests instead of themselves actively engaging in beneficial amounts and kinds of physical activity.

*A Counter Movement Intrudes.* In the meantime, golf courses, tennis courts, the miniature golf fad, bowling, Little League, Boy and Girl Scouts' and Camp Fire Girls' programs, SCUBA- and skin-diving, waterskiing, fishing, out-board motor boating, recreational vehicles, parks, playfields, public and private pools are examples of some organized facilities and other provisions for attracting individuals and families to become participants. This trend began even as it appeared that we were destined to become a nation of "idle watchers." No one could have imagined that the less-than-promising beginnings of the 1920s and 1930s would mushroom into vast amounts of participation in the next fifty years. At the college level, the intramural athletic program began as "pickup" teams of students competed. Later, vast facilities were needed to meet the demand for such participation. The Outdoor Life movement began in a similar way—by unnoticed hikers, bicyclists, mountain-climbers, sports fishermen, nature-lovers, and an occasional car or truck owner propelling his family-laden vehicle to the end of a dirt road.

*The Impact of the World Wars.* One of the factors in the 1920s which led to the increase in an interest in sports as spectator or performer was the public announcement by the armed services of the proportion of rejectees for military service during World War I. Most of the states lacked legislation requiring physical education in the schools and public colleges. Now they passed such laws. Few of these were adequate in provisions for time, proper programs or standards of teacher preparation.

And, few of the causes for rejection were related to physical education, exercise, athletics or the dance. It is not without significance that during World War II no improvement in the "physical condition" of potential inductees over those of WW I was found. Again, almost all the causes for rejection in WW II were unrelated to physical education.

Following World War I, as sometimes has followed other major wars, personal conduct and social and moral standards softened. This became the seed of permissiveness by parents in child-rearing which continues today. The doctrine of relativism in ethics paralleled what appears to be unconcern by many in ethical ideals and standards in the conduct and participation in some sports.

Also related to the spurt in interest in sports following WW I came the commercial "take-over" of an exercise fad as illustrated by health spas, muscle-builders, spot-reducing, feature articles in the press on exercise by Hollywood "names," and books and pamphlets by others equally uninformed.

Women, too, continued to expand their programs, facilities, and professional organizations at local and national levels. Such activities as the following were offered beginning with the 1920s and 1930s: fencing, field hockey, tennis, volleyball, soccer, track and field, skating, archery, equitation, baseball, clog-dancing, interpretive dancing, Natural dancing, stunts and boating including sailing. In addition, extramurals, sports days, play days and telegraphic meets in suitable sports continued to be held. These kept alive the idea of competition in sports between women performers during a time when the value of such was questioned by some of the women leaders in college physical education.

By the time of the Great Depression, recreational programs had begun to develop and enjoy not only popularity but improved organization and supervision. In addition to some of the organizations referred to above, such as the Girl and Boy Scouts, the Playground and Recreation Association of America was formed. Its programs proved helpful during the Depression and the latter prompted the government to increase opportunities for public-supported recreation. These programs revealed the unpreparedness of children and youth to engage in many active forms of recreation. Later, during World War II, young women and men illustrated their possession of skills and desire for participating in active recreational activities. The schools and colleges had learned that one value to which they could contribute, formerly overlooked, was preparing youth for leisure-time programs. The recreational programs paralleled the acceptance and spread of the idea of including some co-educational activities in school and college physical education programs.

Such emphases accentuated the values related to the improvement of the individual as a member of a social group. And, the individual of that day wanted to be in such physical condition, possess such skills, develop a figure or body build that would aid him in being an accepted and popular member of a group. In a wartime setting such values as endurance, stamina and physical fitness came to the fore without difficulty.

Previous to and after World War II college men physical educationalists were concerned with developing safety in sports. Attention was given not only to physical condition but also to equipment, rules, officiating and health examinations in intramurals, intercollegiate and interscholastic athletics. These precautions had been taken previously in the women's programs.

During World War II, there were many attempts to fashion high school programs with a view to enabling women to be in better condition at the time of military induction. In addition, even elementary school playgrounds were cluttered with obstacle courses, cargo-nets and other war-training equipment. In spite of the intentions of these programs, during the war the new inductees did not show improved physical fitness, as measured by the tests of the various military branches.

Following World War II, in spite of the threats of the "Cold War," interest in personal physical condition sharply decreased. In fact, physical education came under attack in schools and colleges. There were many educators and students who opposed the requirement of taking classes in games, sports, exercise and the dance. During this period the Krause-Weber Test was given to a few thousand American children. The resulting scores, as compared with scores of European children, were not favorable to American children. The issue became acute. The result was a conference on *all-around* fitness called by the President of the United States. The next president limited a similar effort to *physical* fitness for *youth*. A similar program was favored by his successor. In the meantime, a federal Council on Physical Fitness for Youth was formed. The results of these efforts have been varied, depending upon the effectiveness of the contributory efforts made at the state and local levels. In states undertaking programs of physical fitness with vigor and enthusiasm, school physical education programs tended to become physical fitness programs, with other values often unaccounted for. A few national organizations supported physical fitness programs. Other professional organizations have continued to emphasize and support a more balanced program, augmenting the physical conditioning feature with games, sports and the dance.

During and after World War II the chief value of physical education was the preservation of the nation. This value continued for some years because of the "Cold" War, in spite of indifference on the part of the general citizenry and many educators. But a return to interest in sports for sports' sake, and continued interest in recreational activities, with an able assist by feature articles in the press, plus a carryover from war years of veterans' personal interest in individual self-image, led to an increase in an "aesthetic emphasis" in the "dance" and, dance as an art form, "body control," "safety," "skillfulness" in popular forms of exercise, "emotional and social growth" of children through play activities, "increased interest in knowledge" of the human body, a "better understanding of self and one's potentials," and some concern over deteriorating ethical standards.

Perhaps the most distinguishing difference between the nineteenth century and the twentieth century in overall value of physical education, the dance and athletics was that in the former, the basic value was the contribution of these activities to education. In the twentieth century, the overall value has been a gradually developing focus on the needs of children and youth. In spite of this, too many educators still (to quote a famous doctor of medicine) ". . . think forty little minds sit in a classroom and forget that they are housed in forty little bodies."

All pertinent scientific facts point to the biological and sociopsychological needs of children and youth for adequate amounts and suitable kinds of muscular activity. Barring pathological conditions, this means that some of this activity must be vigorous. Strength, endurance, speed and most of the biological outcomes do not come without a price. Keeping the physiochemical processes, such as chemical expenditure and restoration, flexible and well-adjusted; and the conditioning of the cardio-respiratory process, are examples of biological values that do not come without a price. This price is imposed by way of beneficial intensities, kinds and amounts of physical activity. Therein lies one prime value. The same goes for beneficial rates and kinds of growth and development of children—resiliencies, densities and responsivenesses of the vital organs.

*"New" Values.* There are "styles" in values related to physical activities, just as there are styles in medicine, architecture and religion. Beginning, roughly, in the 1950s and even before, it was the style to follow the prior lead of T. D. Wood, M.D., Clark Hetherington and Jesse F. Williams, M.D., and their emphases on sociopsychological and moral values attendant on participation in physical activities. Long before, Homer and later Greeks had set the style of attaching religious and aesthetic values to their sports participation, and King Cyrus had set the style of military values connected with the program of exercises and sports for his vast armies.

Basic values of a culture, in spite of their so-called "permanence" do change, if enough beliefs within that culture change sufficiently for a long enough period of time, and with some degree of conviction. Or, at times, a culture's basic values undergo some revision because *many* small values are changed by enough people for a great enough time period. Possible "new" values will emerge for participants in physical activities as the sciences, sociology, psychology, aesthetics and other appropriate fields uncover "new" desired outcomes which today are not discernible. Researches in physiology, kinesiology, biochemistry, sports medicine appear to be the kinds of fields most promising in "new" biological values.

Still another way of searching for "new" values is to consider the chief values of American culture and then to see which of these may be gained at least in part by means of participation in physical activities. This kind of effort was made by Catherine L. Allen (1) at the time she was president of the American Association of Health, Physical Education and Recreation in 1964–65. The committee appointed to this task identified ten chief values in American culture. Five of these were presented in Chapter 2 (page 15). The ten chief values may be broken down into a total of over one hundred subvalues some of which are: self-responsibility, personal health, character development, development of skill, creativity, emotional control, team-play, the Golden Rule, getting along with others, tolerance, sportsmanship, equal rights, fair play, moral decency, desirable outcomes of work at home and school, desirable outcomes and services of recreation and public health, good citizenship, leisure-time skills, personal fitness, appreciation of and involvement in the aesthetic, consideration of and for the rights of others, concern and care for others, helping others meet life's problems, preparation for vocation, harmony among neuro-muscular coordinations, grace of movement, balance and control during performance, enjoyment, pride in personal appearance, lessening of friction among groups, rendering of justice, improvement of education and changes toward improvement in the American way.

The above representative samplings of the subvalues which emerge from an analysis of the principal values of American culture are illustrative of an easily-overlooked phenomenon. Chief values of a going culture (the ways of life and living of a people) are the result of a *synthesis* of those ways of living of *individuals* which have proved best for the development and improvement of humans, under prevading conditions over a consider-able period of time. These values are geared almost always to those life-styles which have proved to be good to and for the persons genuinely and positively involved in that culture. Thus, (1) the *purposes* man sets for himself and his fellows to seek and accomplish, and, (2) the *needs* which he feels must be satisfied and fulfilled, constitute almost all of the "things" that are considered to be good to and for man-in-his-culture. These two operations lead to man's finding sounder evidence supporting his values, to his finding "new" values, and his modifying or jettisoning familiar values which have lost their pertinence.

In this whole process, if both the individual and his culture are to be nurtured and improved upon, man must have and use adequate mental ability to translate his personal and short-range values into the culture's principal and long-range values. He must also have and use his other abilities—physical, moral, emotional, esthetic and spiritual—so that they also contribute to this nurturing and improving process. These comments imply that in a democracy, opportunities and ways exist which enable "new" values to arise and be considered. The "new" value will have such worth and be of such help in furthering human life that it becomes not only a part of the culture's chief values, but may also expand into a chief value.

Yet, even in a democracy, the earnest social experimenter must possess not only the concept of a "new" value but also persistent patience, as well as ideas of how and where it will fit into the culture's hierarchy of values. Further, the "new" value must have affirmative impact on and acceptance by peoples in many walks of life. One of Mortimer Adler's six essential conditions regarding philosophy is that it becomes a *public* enterprise.

The social experimenter also might note the history of his progenitors who also tried to inculcate and promulgate "new" values in a culture. Among other things, he will find that most of those who were unsuccessful in that endeavor caught the "philosopher's contagious disease," namely, selecting and attacking as adversaries those who held differing views, who pursued differing activities and who assigned differing emphases. This "ailment" accounts in large part for the slow march of philosophy from the times of Pythagoras to the present time. In contrast, scientists avoid this "adversary" way of thinking and doing. Ways of doing things, if they are intended to achieve the same goals, can be delightfully different.

One question, one challenge is: to which of the culture's chief values and subvalues can and do physical education, the dance and athletic sports contribute? The answer to that question must be qualified by and yet must overcome two inescapable conditions. *First*, Americans have in their possession vast quantities of leisure time. *Second*, we follow a sedentary pattern of life, watching others perform, or we ride in automobiles, recreational vehicles or motor boats. True, they may carry us to the great outdoors, but it appears that it is these *transportation machines* that "enjoy" the activity, as they whisk us restlessly from one geographic spot to another. Yet, never before have biological values been so needed in physical and mental health, preventive medicine and personal living.

## REFERENCES

1. Allen, Catherine L.; Davis, E. C.; Lynn, Minnie L.; and Wallis, Earl. Report on the President's Committee on "The Significance of the Profession in American Culture," *Journal of Health, Physical Education, Recreation,* November-December 1964, pp. 37–43.

2. Ballou, Ralph B. "An Analysis of the Writings of Selected Church Fathers to A.D. 394 to Reveal Attitudes Regarding Physical Activities." Ph.D. dissertation, University of Oregon, 1965.

3. Ceram, C. W. *The March of Archaeology.* New York: Alfred A. Knopf, 1968, pp. 63–64.

4. Dulles, Foster Rhea. *A History of Recreation.* 2d ed. New York: Meredith Publishing Co., 1965, pp. 22–66.

5. Frankfort, Henri et al. *Before Philosophy.* Baltimore: Penguin Books, 1968, p. 10.

6. Hackensmith, C. W. *History of Physical Education.* New York: Harper & Row Publishers, 1966, pp. 81–126.

7. Ibid., pp. 311–45.

8. Van Dalen, D. B., and Bennett, Bruce. *A World History of Physical Education.* Englewood Cliffs, N.J.: Prentice-Hall, 1971, pp. 365–427.

9. Ibid., pp. 69–126.

10. Ibid., pp. 428–511.

## READINGS

Dulles, Foster Rhea. *A History of Recreation.* 2d ed. New York: Meredith Publishing Co., 1965.

Durant, Will. *The Reformation.* New York: Simon & Schuster, 1955.

Hackensmith, C. W. *History of Physical Education.* New York: Harper & Row Publishers, 1966.

Smith, Preserved. *A History of Modern Culture.* New York: Holt, Rinehart and Winston, 1964.

———. *The Enlightenment: 1687–1776.* New York: Collier Book Co., 1962.

Van Dalen, D. B., and Bennett, Bruce L. *A World History of Physical Education.* Englewood Cliffs, N.J.: Prentice-Hall, 1971.

# 5 | Integration of Biologic Values With a Personal Value System

CIVILIZATION'S BEGINNINGS were made possible, in part, and continued by means of beliefs in and practice of physical activity as something which was useful to man—was good for man—was good to man. Without his knowing about values, early man placed value upon engaging in physical activities.

## BIOLOGIC VALUES AND MAN'S HERITAGE

Modern man may join the anthropologist as he views the role that physical activity played in the cultures of man. Through this medium, man of antiquity carved on stone or clay tablet, leaf and wall his thoughts in poetry, prose and pictograph. By means of muscular activity he explored the land; turned the potter's wheel; crafted tools and weapons; painted, molded, and sculpted. He built thatched huts and erected massive stone monuments. He planted, tilled, and harvested the soil. He built ships and pushed their prows into the unknown.

More specifically, he ran, climbed, leaped, pushed, grappled, pulled, threw, crept, twisted, caught, struck, thrust, tossed, crawled, lifted, clawed, carried, swung, walked, kicked, fell and got up—all a part of his participation in the life of war, worship, work and recreation. His physiology and anatomy set limits as he pursued his purposes, whims, curiosities and met demands.

No one knows to what extent and for how long *Homo sapiens*, *Homo faber* or *Homo ludens* engaged in such age-old activities. We believe today that it is *normal* for man to enjoy physical activity. Such a belief springs not only from racial and personal experiences, but also from the conclusions of the modern psychologist, the biologist and philosopher. What is it that drives members of the animal kingdom to be active, and then for *Homo sapiens*, at least, to find satisfaction during activity of the body? Something happens to the body, its systems, its parts, its functions and its very tissues and cells, during physical activity. Something also seems to happen to unidentified, inner feelings even as man anticipates engaging in some activity. If it is a favorite activity, these feelings are quite unlike those resulting from anticipating an activity that is feared or thoroughly disliked! He also is motivated to involve his whole being.

Most psychologists, considering the fundamental nature of physical activity in life and living, regard physical activity as one of the great motives of man. They also estimate that no child attains normal development and growth without having engaged in beneficial kinds, amounts, intensities and continuities of physical activity. Equal intensity of conviction regarding the value of regular exercise for the normal person comes from the medical profession. *No field has ever produced facts or near-facts contradicting such generalizations.*

Modern man with his science thus joins his precursor, who was furthered only by his guess and untested experience, in the conclusion that physical activity is valuable to and for man.

A strong body of values may be characterized not only as "well-established" and "well-organized," but also augmented by high value placed by the individual on those things that really count *in the long run* and which are *retained under stress*. This, of course, does not mean they should not be open to examination, to scrutiny and to change—if this means the betterment of man, and of society.

Values are highly individual, particularly as the person weaves them into his own life-style and system of values. The individual's hierarchy of values depends greatly on his experiences and judgment. His selection of values depends also on his reaction to life's experiences. Further, it depends on what he *does* about his reactions. There are some large-scale values which are held by almost all members of a group, a nation, a civilization.

The beginnings of some of today's values are rooted deeply in lessons learned by prethinking man. Similarly, one can understand some of today's basic values of American culture as he studies life in the colonial and early-nation periods of this country and that in the native countries of immigrants, as we have seen.

There may be relationships between these individual and collective views of values, and, certain considerations of early animal life. For example, there are the suggestions of Pierre Teilhard de Chardin in his brilliant *The Phenomenon of Man* that there was *choice* long before pre-thinking man. Many biologists conjecture that even simple forms of life make choices in terms of reacting to heat, light, colors, odors and the like. There appears to be some basis for thinking that man's making choices may be a part of a continuum of choice-making through the panorama of animal life. Some biologists hazard the guess that even very simple forms of animal life choose ways that result in their survival. It is hypothesized that refinements, such as reacting in ways that brought comfort or the avoidance of discomfiture or pain, were gradually added. The basis of preferences began somehow, somewhere.

As objectionable as these conjectures may be to biologists with contrary opinions, it seems reasonable to take the view that some values held by most men today stem from age-old experiences and hoary conclusions of the ancients as they met and reacted to life's goodness and woe, and to the impact of experiences.

*Responsibility and Consequences.*   Whatever the source of values and whatever the vehicle by means of which the individual gains, assigns or sees values, that person *cannot avoid being responsible for the consequences,* come as they may. It is *one's own* judgment that is involved in choosing values and in identifying their source(s). It is true that a number of forces play upon him, influencing his choice of values. His own prejudices, emotions, wants and attitudes also influence his choice of decisions.

More profoundly, the culture of which the individual is a part as a rule sets the *general* style and taste in many values for its members. Nevertheless, it is the person himself who selects the values that comprise his own value system. He must live with the consequences of this system. He must live with the consequences of the attitudes he permits himself, until and unless changes are made in his beliefs, his value-system, in the culture or in his attitudes.

Responsibility is emphasized here for two reasons. *First,* many individuals rationalize their behavior without ever connecting it with their value systems. Behavior stems from beliefs. People do not do all that they believe, but whatever they do springs from some belief, particularly those things which are linked to values. *Second,* even though values prove inadequate, this does not mean that the unfortunate consequences are to be endured forever. It is as simple as it is difficult to do, if one is to escape the consequences. *We modify unsatisfactory values or adopt new ones*—or suffer the consequences unnecessarily.

*Modern Concern About Values.* There appears to be widening national concern about values. People more than vaguely sense it—they seem to know it. They discuss troublesome matters which rest directly on values and their interpretations. Works of art, music and literature may be or may reflect protests against disvalue and hollowness in some facets of daily living.

The peoples of both experienced and awakening nations are forcing Americans to look at themselves—inwardly and outwardly. We, like other humans, tend *to not think* until we have to, until we are in pain or suffer discomfort. What does one find as he examines the American scene—the American public—himself? What of his inner fiber, character, enduring values? What does the foreign observer think of the sincerity of American humanitarianism when he sees American materialism in operation? As he reads American novels? As he sees American movies? As he observes the "typical" American tourist? As he visits American cities? As he senses our values? Our *biological* values?

Part of the national concern about values is geared inescapably to apprehension about the condition of the biological self. The American's work, well-being, vitality, health, zest, leisure activities are linked partly to physical activity and its outcomes. Is the current neglect of the biological by some Americans a result of ignorance of consequences? If not, what is it?

*Agreement and Disagreement on Values.* Biologically and socially similar people place different degrees and kinds of values on identical objects, ideas, things, experiences. Yet at least a few gross dissimilarities exist in values of those who come from similar backgrounds, socioeconomic-educational levels, and enjoy similar ways of life. The most obvious example of this paradox is found within a given national culture where basic values typify the life-style of the people, yet within the nation are noteworthy individual exceptions, sometimes referred to as *regional* values.

In spite of efforts to educate tastes and preferences, humans differ in what they *permit* life to do to their emotions, motives, attitudes, and the rest, that is, each man *lives* differently. He *interprets* life differently. All this is by way of saying that regardless of the events and the environment, some men agree and other men disagree on even large-scale values.

There are of course some things that most men do feel are values.

Some things they feel are disvalues (1): being a traitor; being disloyal to one's kind; being untrustworthy; being treacherous; being cruel to the weak, crippled and sick; being hollow in character; being easily angered; being unjust; and being disrespectful toward man.

*Values Divide and Unify Men.*   Even the acknowledged over-simplification of the foregoing discussion is sufficient to permit the conclusion that values are both divisive *and* unifying forces. Acts of disloyalty, political party splits, quarrels, upheavals within any organization, as well as wars and religious schisms, are basically the result of differences in values among men. There are not only differences as to things upon which value is placed, differences in degrees of value assigned to a given thing, differences in the kinds of value which are the most important; there are also differences as to the nature of value and its source(s).

Nevertheless, there is equal evidence supporting the observation that values motivate men to friendliness, to a meeting of minds, to the establishment of peace, to amicability, to conciliation, to interpersonal adjustment, to cooperation, and to other sorts of unity.

Large-scale values, such as the physical welfare of people, are particularly powerful in bringing men together in thought and action. Students of value (axiologists) vehemently disagree on many details within their field, but they unite solidly when it comes to the value of studying value! Professors, students and parents may disagree on some of the details of education, but they unite on its value as a social institution. Thus, looked at in the large—broadly—and in the long run, *values often tend to unite men.* Looked at in the *small*—narrowly—values often tend to divide men.

*Conflicting Values.*   Experiencing conflicts within one's hierarchy of values is no longer an unusual occurrence in an increasingly complex society. To consider the power of values in no way eliminates the presence of conflict in values. The individual who must decide between a good and an evil thing may find the decision difficult, but this often does not begin to compare with the difficulty of deciding between two good things. The element of confusion in the latter is, initially, an ever-present possibility.

Most of the opposition to engaging in exercise usually is not a denial of the values of physical activity. Rather, it often is a case of a conflict of these values with those associated with some other enterprise that also seems worthy. But, *this fact does not enable the student to escape the consequences.*

There probably is a good deal of wasted time, thought and effort over the question of the values of physical activity. When carefully examined, there is no case against *beneficial* kinds, amounts, intensities and continuities of physical activity. The usual disagreement is over whether this activity is good for man as an *end* in itself, or as *leading on* to something else which is of *value* to the individual.

Someone has pointed out that in any aspect of life that demands percepto-motor skill, the performer does more than make selections and reselections of his neurosensory mechanisms. He strives for some goal(s). He may have the joy of attaining it. He experiences the satisfactions that accompany engaging in physical activity, the satisfaction of moving, of using his muscles. Often he experiences that vague but real feeling of "self-realization" and "self-fulfillment." This general thought is companion to the ". . . *sheer harmony of its* (the body's) *properly functioning organs* gives us a flood of unconscious enjoyment . . ." that A. N. Whitehead, Harvard's eminent philosopher, talked about while being interviewed by Lucien Price, during forty-three dialogues with this eminent Harvard philosopher.

### BIOLOGIC VALUES AND THE INDIVIDUAL'S SYSTEM OF VALUES

As the next five chapters present and discuss the large-scale biological values of physical activity, what are the chances that those values will become activated within one's life style? For the young adult who is fortunate enough to be free from pathological conditions, all biological values may play a role in his system of values and therefore in his day-to-day living. But, carrying that statement into action demands something more than reading about it, possessing this knowledge, knowing the supporting facts or observing the changes in energy, health and enjoyment of other persons. One aid to practicalizing values is to *weave them into* one's personal system of values.

Many possible values, related to physical activity in many of its forms, have been presented in the previous chapters. They form a vast reservoir from which one might choose values or that might lead to values more suitable to the individual's own life-style. Chapter 2 presented a dozen aspects of life which are suggestive of "parts" of one's life to which one might expect to attach values. Some of these relate to physical activity. Chapter 2 also presents some of the sources of personal values, in addition to some steps and tests useful in selecting values. Such aids apply directly to biological values.

It is suggested that *purposely* selecting values, being aware of their significance and their source, as well as of some of the difficulties involved, is in the direction of being knowledgeable in this value-selection process, a first step in formulating a system of values that not only fits one's present life-style, but also influences it. Thus, one is supported and strengthened not only in what values he already has, but also in his methods of acquiring new values. Without some such organized approach, he wears "blinders" in his value-selection. Another organized approach to forming a system of values is suggested by beginning with large-scale values, analyzing them so that detailed values emerge and then to examine these latter in terms of the quality of their sources, with searching questions as to their applicability to life and one's life-style.

## REFERENCES

1. Clough, Shepard B. *Basic Values of Western Civilization*. New York: Columbia University Press, 1960.

## READINGS

Cowell, Charles C., and France, Wellman L. *Philosophy and Principles of Physical Education*. Englewood Cliffs, N.J.: Prentice-Hall, 1963.

Davis, Elwood Craig, ed. *Philosophies Fashion Physical Education*. Dubuque, Iowa: Wm. C. Brown Co., 1963.

de Chardin, Pierre Teilhard. *The Phenomenon of Man*. New York: Harper & Row Publishers, 1964.

Dubos, René. *The Torch of Life*. New York: Pocket Books, 1963.

———. *Man Adapting*. New Haven: Yale University Press, 1967.

———. *The Dreams of Reason, Science and Utopias*. New York: Columbia University Press, 1961.

Durant, Will. *The Pleasures of Philosophy*. New York: Simon and Schuster, 1953.

Fromm, Erich. *Man For Himself*. New York: Holt, Rinehart and Co., 1960.

Gagne, Robert H., and Fleishman, Edwin A. *Psychology and Human Performance*. New York: Henry Holt and Co., 1959.

*Goals for Americans*. Englewood Cliffs, N.J.: Prentice-Hall, 1964.

Heard, Gerald. *The Five Ages of Man*. New York: Julian Press, 1963.

Hook, Sidney. *Dimensions of the Mind*. New York: Collier Books (BS38), 1964.

Huizinga, Jan. *Homo Ludens*. London: Routledge and Kegan Paul, 1959.

Maslow, Abraham. *New Knowledge of Human Values*. New York: Harper & Brothers, 1959.

Matthias, Eugen. *The Deeper Meaning of Physical Education*. New York: A. S. Barnes & Co., 1929.

McCloy, Charles H. *Philosophical Bases for Physical Education*. New York: F. S. Crofts & Co., 1940.

Mumford, Lewis. *The Conduct of Life.* New York: Harcourt, Brace, Jovanovich, Inc., 1970.

Murphy, Gardner. *Human Potentialities.* New York: Basic Books, Inc., 1958.

Price, Lucian. *Dialogues of Alfred North Whitehead.* Boston: Little, Brown & Co., 1956.

Report of the President's Committee on "The Significance of the Profession in American Culture." *Journal of Health, Physicial Education, Recreation,* November-December, 1964, pp. 37–43.

Tyrell, G. N. M. *Homo Faber.* London: Methuen & Co., 1951.

White, Morton, ed. *The Age of Analysis: 20th Century Philosophers.* New York: The New American Library (Mentor MT 353), 1955.

Whyte, Lancelot Law. *The Next Development in Man.* New York: The New American Library, 1950.

# PART 3

## Biologic Adaptations and Physical Activity

**OVERVIEW**   Physical activity is directly related to the structure and function of the human body. Major body tissues and organs are modified through the stimulus of muscular activity. Thus, bodily proportions can be changed by a long-term regimen of exercise. Normal growth and development are related to regular physical activity stress. Internally, the major physiological systems respond both acutely and chronically to exercise. The changes in the cardiovascular, respiratory, nervous and metabolic systems are related to improved physiological efficiency and to the possible prevention of certain chronic disease entities. Such scientifically determined results are seen as facts that support the possibility of one's gaining biological values from engaging in physical activity.

# 6 | Morphophysiological Adaptations to Muscular Activity

LOGIC INHERENTLY leads one to the supposition that, biologically, man possesses an innate need to move. Morphophysiology deals with the physiological processes which control the growth and development processes and changes in body morphology or organ structure. And, muscular activity, to be sure, does provide an important stimulus to the normal growth and development process. This accounts for the natural propensity for vigorous physical activity in the rapidly developing child and adolescent. Invariably, children deprived of normal opportunity for physical activity lack proper physical development and are smaller in physical stature than their peers (19).

## SKELETAL RESPONSE TO ACTIVITY

Although it has been well demonstrated that the growth and development process is generally under the control of the anterior pituitary hormone (somatotrophin) and influenced by other variables such as heredity, climate, diet and disease entities, it is also moderated through exercise (6). Experimental studies of animals placed in movement-deprived environments (as, for example, crowded cages) indicate that they do not achieve their normal species growth potential and die at a relatively early age. Much more study, however, is needed in order to describe more definitively the relationship between children's opportunity for physical activity and the changing nature of the growth processes. It seems logical to assume that the physical stimulus of exercise would be most important during the rapid growth periods (such as the preschool years and the prepuberty growth spurt) because of the recognized physiological relationship between structure and function.

Wolff first outlined the applications of the structure function principle to skeletal growth (1). In essence, Wolff held that changes in bony growth or configuration were brought about in part by externally imposed mechanical stress. Knipping and Valentin (13) later referred more specifically to the "kinetic stress or stimulus" and emphasized its importance to optimal growth and function of the bones and musculature. Generally, it appears that bone, muscle tissue, and certain other connective tissues respond structurally (with changes in anatomic configuration) and in quality of function in direct response to the imposed mechanical demands placed upon them. Specific examples of this are outlined below.

It was first noted in 1933 in cadaver studies of athletes that they had developed a more massive and dense skeleton than nonathletes (25). Other studies demonstrated that athletes develop larger bony protuberances at the points of attachment for ligaments and tendons. Structures on the surface of the bone which are not stressed may disappear and new bone particles (trabeculae) may develop when new mechanical stresses require increased stability for the adhering connective tissue (3).

Recently, Buskirk et al. (5) compared X-rays of the forearms and hands of a group of nationally ranked tennis players and a group of nontennis players which displayed slight increases in length of the radius and ulna in the dominant arm and an increase in breadth in the distal end of the ulna. They also found that the tennis players had a much greater development of the bones and muscles in the dominant arm as compared to the nondominant arm. In studies where subjects are immobilized in a supine position in bed for many weeks, the skeletal system begins to demineralize and large amounts of calcium are lost in the urine (25, 21). This mineral breakdown and softening of the bone is not caused solely by loss of gravity stress on the skeletal system but more particularly by lack of mechanical exercise stress. This was ascertained after some of the subjects were allowed to sit up rather than maintain the recumbent position for the period of experimentally forced inactivity (21). These studies have many implications for the maintenance of good skeletal function and mechanically efficient posture.

### MUSCLE RESPONSE TO ACTIVITY

Morpurgo (15) and Siebert (23) demonstrated many years ago that muscle tissue shows a morphophysiological response to exercise stress which is similar to that of bone. Specific kinds of exercise stress will produce a morphological response known as muscle hypertrophy (increase in muscle bulk). This muscular hypertrophy response is quite evident in individuals who have participated for many years in high resistance muscular activity. It has been well demonstrated that the increases in muscle size which occur as a result of repeated mechanical stress (e.g., weight training) are due primarily to an enlargement of the already existing fibers. These individual fibers show an increase in cross sectional diameter and its protoplasmic constituent (sarcoplasm).

Several experimenters (14, 20) working with animals have published results which indicate that prolonged training may create a small number of new muscle fibers (hyperplasia). If prolonged training does produce such hyperplastic changes it is assumed to be minimal and representative of only a small proportion of the total hypertrophy which transpires. With disuse of muscle tissue there is a decline in the contractile protein myofibrils, an increase in the fat content of the muscle, and overall loss of size referred to as atrophy (7). Several investigators have shown that training for muscular endurance produces an increase in the number of capillaries supplying a given area of muscle tissue (25, 18). Training may also aid increased blood flow to muscle tissue by stimulating the development of new blood vessels, called collaterals, which open only during exercise stress (22).

## CONNECTIVE TISSUE RESPONSE TO ACTIVITY

In addition to the biological adaptations which occur in bone and muscle tissue as a function of muscular activity, similar adaptations have been noted in the various connective tissue. Holmdahl and Ingelmark (8) recently showed that exercised animals develop thicker articular cartilage in their joints than unexercised controls. This joint cartilage serves as a buffer between bony surfaces in the joint and helps to protect the joint against injury. That exercise provides a significant functional stress for cartilaginous tissue was demonstrated by ten minutes of running, bringing about a 12–13 percent increase in its thickness, presumably brought about by fluid absorption (11). Such absorption and thickening should significantly increase the buffering or shock absorption function of the cartilage during exercise stress. For this reason, warm-up activities should include progressive exercise of those joints which may be stressed during participation in subsequent vigorous activity.

Several researchers (2, 10, 27, 28) have presented evidence regarding an increase in the size and tensile strength of the ligaments and tendons as a result of longterm imposition of mechanical stress on these tissues through the medium of physical activity. This change in size and strength is brought about by increased formation of both elastic and nonelastic protein fibers which make up the connective tissue and also the chemical ground substance or cement which binds the tissue together (9). Since the ligament is proportionately the weakest of the connective tissue and, therefore, most susceptible to trauma, longitudinal conditioning programs should provide for progressive graded stress of this tissue well before any participation in all-out body contact sports activities which might result in trauma to the connective tissue.

### CHANGES IN BODY COMPOSITION

Conditioning activities which are of significantly high caloric expenditure can, over a period of several months, significantly influence total body weight and the quality of the body composition. The popular dictum that you have to exercise too hard and too long to significantly affect body weight is no longer substantiated by scientific study. Mayer's (16) review of studies in this area with both animals and humans substantiates that there is a cumulative caloric value inherent in regular exercise that is often misunderstood by the average layman who is unsophisticated in metabolic physiology. That is, although a single bout of exercise is of little metabolic significance the repetition of that bout three times per week over a period of many months will have a profound effect on the balance of the human metabolic processes. For example, fifteen minutes of jogging will expend only about 350 calories in the average size man. This is less calories than that ingested in a light lunch. If the same individual, however, jogs 3 days in one week he has expended over 1000 calories, and in one month's time over 4000 calories, which is in excess of the normal food intake for one day.

Over a period of many months, or one year, regular exercise can be the difference between maintenance of ideal body weight rather than succumbing to the problem of creeping overweight. Life insurance actuarial statistics show that the average American gains slightly less than 1 pound per year after reaching physiological maturity (late teens or early twenties).

When combined with a mild dietary restriction program regular vigorous physical activity offers a most efficient and safe means of weight reduction. Optimum activities for this purpose are those emphasizing endurance, such as running, bicycling, swimming, and so on. Principles of endurance training are presented in Chapter 10. Muscular activity can also be used most effectively for maintaining normative body weight once that goal has been achieved. Theoretically, a person with a normal metabolism (i.e., absence of thyroid imbalance) could eat as much as he wanted if he were willing to exercise strenuously enough on a regular basis. The importance of high metabolic expenditure activity is enlarged when one considers the high relationship between obesity and cardiovascular disease, particularly hypertension (12). It may well be that the most important preventive role of exercise in coronary heart disease is an indirect one, through the control of body weight and excess body fat.

Several body composition studies (4, 17, 24, 30) point to the value of vigorous activity in reducing the relative proportion of body fat to other tissue. It is not unusual for adults to reduce their percent body fat by as much as two percent in just ten weeks of regular participation (three times weekly) in jogging activities (30). This decrease in body fat is usually associated with a moderate increase in muscle tissue (3). Muscle tissue is relatively dense and therefore tends to partially offset the body weight loss achieved through fat decrease. The change in the body's proportion of muscle tissue as a function of exercise is designated physiologically as lean body mass. This lean body mass increase is significant from a physiological point of view and cannot be measured from simple determinations of body weight at various points in the conditioning program. This means that changes in total body weight cannot be used to evaluate the metabolic efficacy of a conditioning program. Such a measure provides only a gross quantitative assessment and provides no information regarding qualitative changes in the body tissue. To ascertain qualitative changes in the body tissue (i.e., lean body mass and percent body fat) it is necessary to utilize laboratory body composition techniques.

There are two basic laboratory methods for the measurement of body composition. In Figures 6.1 and 6.2 changes in percent body fat are estimated from several skin fold measurements at various anatomical sites. Figure 6.3 depicts the use of the underwater weighing technique from which lean body mass and percent body fat can be calculated by formula. This is possible since fat has a lower specific gravity and muscle a higher specific gravity than water.

Ideally, individuals would like to differentially reduce the size of the subcutaneous fat pads at various anatomic locations. Unfortunately, there is no conclusive research evidence that fat loss can be localized by exercising a specific body part, sometimes referred to as spot reducing. Apparently, the site of reduction of body fat is determined by the differential size of the fat pads and not by the part of the body exercised. If a person regularly exercises and/or limits his dietary intake sufficiently the metabolization of his fat stores will occur in all of his fat stores. The largest loss will be in the largest fat pads and the least loss in the smallest pads. Or

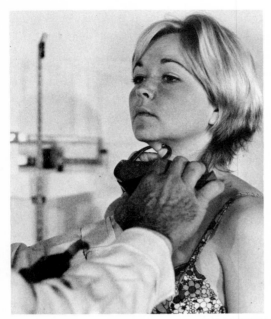

*FIGURE 6.1    Fat Skin Fold Measurement*

*FIGURE 6.2    Fat Skin Fold Measurement*

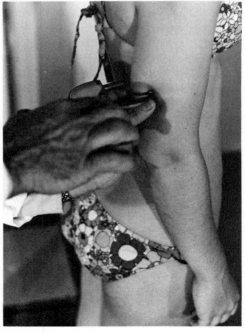

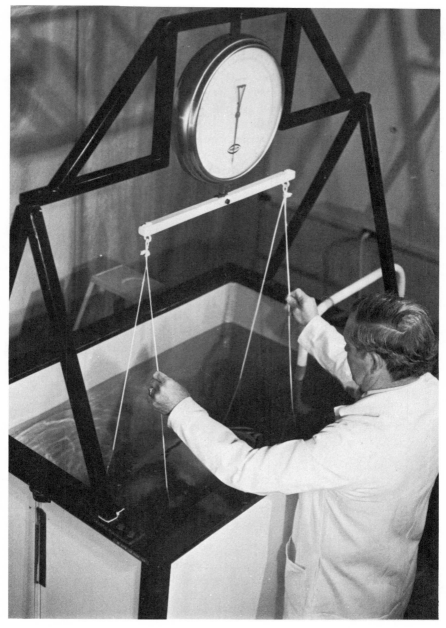

FIGURE 6.3    Body Composition Measurement—Underwater Weighing

expressed in another way, we tend to lose fat proportionately in the various body parts in parallel with the pattern by which it was originally gained, and this is partially a genetically determined variable. Although we cannot localize fat loss by exercising a specific body part, we can use various kinds of exercise stress (such as weight training) to increase local muscle strength, tonus, and mass. By selectively determining which muscle groups we will differentially train we can change our body proportions and overall anatomic configuration.

In our culture the aesthetic appreciation of the well-formed or well-developed body is regarded as a value by many persons. This cultural value parallels that of several other societies and is closely allied to our emphasis on sports and physical fitness. Research on morphophysiological adaptations to muscular activity indicates some of the many benefits to be gained from participation in exercise, sports and the dance. These adaptations are highly specific and are dependent on specialized, regular mechanical stressing of the various body tissues.

## SUMMARY

Morphophysiological processes are moderated by man's opportunity and capacity for movement. Bone and muscle configuration are affected by the mechanical stresses of gross physical activity. The proportions of muscle and fat can be significantly influenced by long term participation in strength and endurance activities and thus total body configuration modified. In addition, exercise causes a thickening and strengthening of the connective tissues (cartilage, ligaments, and tendons) thereby raising the individual's resistance to traumatic injury. Longitudinal participation in vigorous muscular activity results in quantitative and qualitative changes of the total body composition.

## REFERENCES

1. Abramson, Arthur S., and Delagi, Edward F. "The Contributions of Physical Activity to Rehabilitation." *Research Quarterly* 31, no. 2, pt. 2 (May 1960):365.
2. Adams, A. "Effects of Exercise Upon Ligament Strength." *Research Quarterly* 37 (May 1966):2.
3. Astrand, P. O., and Rodahl, K. *Textbook of Work Physiology.* New York: McGraw-Hill, 1970.
4. Behnke, A. R. "Body Composition Studies Relating to Developmental Rate and

Levels of Physical Fitness," Paper presented to the American College of Sports Medicine, March 10, 1967, at Las Vegas.

5. Buskirk, Elsworth R.; Anderson, K. Lange; and Brozek, Joseph. "Unilateral Activity and Bone and Muscle Development in the Forearm." *Research Quarterly* 27, no. 2 (May 1956) :127.

6. Espenchade, Anna. "The Contributions of Physical Activity to Growth." *Research Quarterly* 31, no. 2, pt. 2 (May 1960) :351.

7. Helander, E. "Muscular Atrophy and Lipomorphosis Induced by Immobilizing Plaster Casts." *Acta Morphol. Neerl. Scand.* 3 (1960) :92.

8. Holmdahl, D. E. and Ingelmark, B. E. "Der Bau des Gelenkknorpels unter verschiendenen funktionellen Verhaltnissen." *Acta Anat.* 6 (1948) :309.

9. Inglemark, B. E. "Morphophysiological Aspects of Gymnastic Exercises." *F.I.E.P. Bulletin* 27 (1957) :37–44.

10. Inglemark, B. E. "Der Bau der Schenen wahrend verschiedner Altersperioden und unter wechselnden funktionellen Bedingungen I." *Acta Anat.* 6 (1948) :113.

11. Inglemark, B. E., and Ekholm, R. "A Study on the Variations in the Thickness of Articular Cartilage in Association with Rest and Periodical Load." *Uppsola Lokareforenings Forhandlingar* 5 (1948) :61.

12. Inter Society Commission for Heart Disease Resources, "Primary Prevention of the Atherosclerotic Diseases." *Circulation* 140 (December 1970).

13. Knipping, H. W., and Udentin, H. "Sports In Medicine." In *Therapeutic Exercise,* edited by Sidney Licht. New York: Elizabeth Licht, Publisher, 1961.

14. Longe, B. Van. "The Response of Muscle to Strenuous Exercise." *Journal of Bone and Joint Surgery* 44 (1962) :711.

15. Morpurgo, P. "Uber Aktivitats-Hypertrophie der Willkurlichen Muskeln." *Virchows Arch.* 150 (1897) :522.

16. Mayer, Jean. "Exercise and Weight Control." *Exercise and Fitness.* Chicago: Athletic Institute, 1959.

17. Parizkava, J., and Poupa, O. "Some Metabolic Consequences of Adaptation to Muscular Work." *British Journal of Nutrition* 17 (1963) :341.

18. Petren, T.; Sjostrand, T.; and Sylven, B. "Der Einfluss der Trainings and die Heufigkeit der Capillaren in Herz-und Skelellmuskulatur." *Arbeitphysiol.* 9 (1936) :376.

19. Rarick, G. Laurence. "Exercise and Growth." In *Science and Medicine of Exercise and Sports,* edited by W. R. Johnson. New York: Harper & Brothers, 1960.

20. Reitsma, W. "Regeneratie, Volumertrische en Numerieke Hypertrophie van Skeletspieren bij Kikker en Rat." *Acad. Proefschrift, Vrije Onnersiteit Te Amsterdam.* 1965.

21. Rodahl, K.; Birkhead, N. E.; Blizzard, J. J.; Issekutz, B.; and Pruett, E. D. R. "Physiological Changes during Prolonged Bed Rest." In *Nutrition and Physical Activity,* edited by G. Blix. Stockholm: Almquist and Wiksell, 1967.

22. Schoop, W. "Auswerkungen gesteigerter korperlicher Activitat auf gesunde and krankhaft veranderte Extremitatsarterien." In *Korperliche Aktivitat und Herz und Kreislauferkraukungen,* edited by J. Roskamm et al. Munich: Johann Ambrosius Barth, 1966.

23. Siebert, W. W. "Unlersuchungen uber Hypertrophie des Skelellmuskels." *Z. Klin. Med.* 109 (1929) :350.

24. Skinner, J. S.; Holloszy, K. O.; and Cureton, T. K. "Effects of a Program of Endurance Exercises on Physical Work." *American Journal of Cardiology* 14 (1964) : 747.

25. Steinhaus, A. H. "Chronic Effects of Exercise." *Physiological Reviews* 13 (1933) : 103.

26. Taylor, H. L.; Henschel, A.; Brozek, J.; and Keys, A. "Effects of Bed Rest on Cardiovascular Function and Work Performance." *Journal of Applied Physiology* 2 (1949) :223.

27. Tipton, C. M.; James, S. L.; Mergner, W.; and Tcheng, T. K. "Influence of Exercise on Strength of Medial Collateral Knee Ligaments of Dogs." *American Journal of Physiology* 218 (1970) :894.

28. Vannoti, A., and Pfister, H. "Unlersuchungen Zum Studium des Trainiestseins," *Arbeitsphysiol.* 7 (1934) :127.

29. Viidik, A. "Biomechanics and Functional Adaptations of Tendons and Joint Ligaments." In *Studies on the Anatomy and Function of Bone and Joints* edited by F. G. Evans. Heidelberg: Springer Verlag OHG, 1966.

30. Wilmore, J.; Royce, J.; Guandola, R.; Katch, F.; and Katch, V. "Body Composition Changes with a Ten Week Program of Jogging." *Medicine and Science in Sports* 3 (1970) :113.

# 7 | Internal Physiological Adaptations to Muscular Activity

ALTHOUGH THE term "homeostasis" (milieu interieur) was probably first coined by Cannon, Claude Bernard first described the phenomenon as regulation of the internal environment (20). Despite the wide range of variation that occurs in the external environment, man's internal environment is maintained at a relatively constant biological level until the organism is stressed. The term "relatively constant" is emphasized because most systemic functions normally display considerable variability at rest (6). The normal resting limits or ranges of physiological variability are grossly extended during the stress of exercise.

The physiological modifications which occur in response to exercise stress can be generally categorized as those which are acute or transitory in nature (often referred to as physiological adjustment) and those which are more chronic or long-lasting (often referred to as physiological adaptation). The latter changes are most important to the study of the biological values of muscular activity. They require many weeks or months of exercise training to achieve. Examples of acute adjustments and chronic adaptation to exercise are listed in Table 7.1.

## ACUTE ADJUSTMENTS TO ACTIVITY

Examination of Table 7.1 indicates that the acute or regulatory adjustments to exercise are primarily transitory in nature and represent the

83

TABLE 7.1 Some Examples of Acute and Chronic Adaptations to Muscular Activity

| ACUTE OR REGULATORY PHYSIOLOGICAL ADJUSTMENTS | CHRONIC PHYSIOLOGICAL ADAPTATIONS |
|---|---|
| 1. Increased $O_2$ Consumption | 1. Increased Maximum Work Capacity (Aerobic Capacity) |
| 2. Increased Pulmonary Ventilation and Respiratory Rate | 2. Increased Maximum Oxygen Debt (Anerobic Capacity) |
| 3. Increased Heart Rate | 3. Increased Maximum Cardiac Output |
| 4. Increased Cardiac Output | 4. Increased Maximum Pulmonary Ventilation |
| 5. Increased Systolic Blood Pressure | 5. Increased Heart Volume |
| 6. Increased Body Core Temperature | 6. Lower Resting, Working and Recovery Heart Rates and Blood Pressure |
| 7. Increased Sweat Rate | 7. Increased $O_2$ Extraction by Muscle Tissue |
| 8. Haemoconcentration (increase in red blood cells) | 8. Increased Blood Volume |
| 9. Increased Blood Flow to Skin and Muscles | 9. Increased Levels of Circulating Hemoglobin |
| 10. Decreased Blood Flow to Viscera, Kidney, Bone and Brain | 10. Increased Muscle Girth (Hypertrophy) and Strength |
| 11. Decreased Gastric Mobility and Secretion | 11. Increased Capillarization of Heart and Skeletal Muscle |
| 12. Decreased Urinary Output | 12. Increased Muscle Tissue in Proportion to Fat Tissue (Increase in Lean Body Mass) |
| 13. Decreased Salivary Flow | 13. Increased Flexibility and Strength of Connective Tissue |
| 14. Decreased Plasma Water | 14. Increased Bone Density |
| 15. Complex Changes in Vascular and Cellular Chemistry | 15. Increased Physiological Efficiency and Reserve Capacity |

physiological means by which the body's increased demand for oxygen is supported. As the individual initiates muscular activity the muscle cells begin to metabolize fuel (glucose) at a faster rate to support the increased energy output and this requires many physiological regulatory adjustments. For example, the increased need for oxygen results in an increase in the volume of air being moved by the lungs (pulmonary ventilation) and the breathing rate increases. Blood flow must be increased in order to move the oxygen to the working muscle cells at a faster rate. In addition, increased blood flow during exercise is important for the efficient removal of cell waste products (metabolites) such as carbon dioxide. The blood volume pumped by the heart each minute (cardiac output) increases significantly along with blood pressure. The multiplication of metabolic activity on the part of working muscle cells ($O_2$ consumption processes) results in increased heat production which raises body temperature and induces sweating for purposes of evaporative cooling.

In addition to the above listed regulatory changes, many nonessential physiological functions are inhibited or reduced in scope so as to conserve energy (20). Thus, blood flow to the muscles and skin is increased; blood flow to the viscera, kidneys and brain is reduced. The urinary and digestive functions are almost completely shut down during vigorous activity so as to conserve physiological energy resources.

Most of these acute or immediate responses to exercise return to the pre-exercise or resting level of function within a short period of time after the cessation of activity. How quickly one may recover to his resting level of physiological function is dependent upon the level of activity and his general state of fitness or conditioning. A sedentary person who is acutely stressed with a very high level of exercise may take several hours to physiologically "recover." Such physiological indices as $O_2$ consumption, heart rate, pulmonary ventilation and blood pressure return more quickly to the basal levels in well-conditioned persons. Understanding of this relationship has formed the basis for several tests of physiological fitness.

## CHRONIC ADAPTATIONS TO ACTIVITY

The more long-term adaptations to regular participation in physical activity are listed in the right-hand column of Table 7.1. The degree to which any of these more chronic adaptations to exercise will occur is wholly dependent upon the nature and duration of the physical activity training program. For example, persons training in weightlifting activities do not develop much greater cardiovascular efficiency but do demonstrate increased muscle bulk (hypertrophy) and strength. Conversely, persons participating in vigorous endurance activities (such as running, swimming, bicycling, and the like) will usually not experience much change in muscle bulk but will undergo profound changes in pulmonary and cardiovascular function indicative of significantly improved physiological work efficiency. In other words, the biological adaptations to the stress of exercise are dependent upon the specific nature of the training stimulus.

More specific physiological adaptations to the specific training stimuli of a strength, a flexibility or an endurance conditioning program are presented here in Part 3. Essentially, all of these chronic adaptations to muscular activity provide evidence of an increased physiological reserve capacity on the part of the well-conditioned person. His skeletal and heart muscle, as well as lungs and blood vessels, possess an emergency or reserve quality which permits him to participate in high level physical activity without undue stress being imposed upon his physiological makeup.

Many of the parameters of fitness or biological adaptation are related to one's general physical health. Particular consideration is given to the pulmonary-respiratory, cardiovascular, metabolic and endocrine functions in the remainder of this chapter. Generally speaking, significant adaptations in these physiological functions require relatively high levels of physical activity on a regular basis for several months, and in some instances years of training are required.

*Pulmonary-Respiratory Adaptations.* Since man's exercise or work capacity is primarily limited by his ability to transfer oxygen from the atmospheric air to his working muscle cells, he must move large quantities of air through his lungs. The measure of this function is called minute or pulmonary ventilation and is expressed in liters per minute. Several studies have demonstrated that training results in more economical ventilation during work (*11, 30*). After as little as seven weeks of endurance training the same level of physical work may require 15 percent less minute pulmonary ventilation. This is a change in physiological efficiency which is apparently quickly lost, however, during detraining. Trained athletes demonstrate dramatic ability to achieve very high levels of maximum pulmonary ventilation. After many years of training and adaptation, endurance athletes are able to go from a resting ventilation of 6 liters to over 200 liters per minute (*29*). This kind of adaptation represents remarkable changes in the metabolic and mechanical efficiency of the pulmonary musculature.

In addition to more efficient pulmonary ventilatory function, highly trained athletes can easily transfer oxygen from the alveoli of the lungs into the blood of the lung capillaries (*25*). The increase in this function, which is known as pulmonary diffusing capacity, is probably related in part to genetic predisposition but apparently can be brought about by adherence to a very high level conditioning program. Championship competitive swimmers appear to demonstrate the largest increases in diffusing capacity with training (*24*).

Several studies (*16, 35, 38*) have attributed greater resting lung capacities (vital capacity) to trained athletes, although this is an area of research with contradictory findings (12). Stuart and Collings (35) compared a male sedentary group with a physically active group and after correcting for differences in age, height and weight found significantly higher mean vital capacities in favor of the trained group. These differences undoubtedly represent stronger, more compliant respiratory muscles which are involved in the mechanical control of the breathing maneuver. Since persons who suffer from obstructive lung disease such as tuberculosis and emphysema consistently demonstrate lowered vital capacity, the increased capacity of the trained individual is presumed to be physiologically advantageous (13).

*Cardiovascular Adaptations.* During exercise the lungs are responsible for delivering sufficient quantities of oxygen to the blood to meet the increased metabolic demands of the working muscle cells. Once the circulating pulmonary blood becomes saturated with oxygen the coordinated efforts of the cardiovascular system are required to deliver the oxygen to all of the tissues of the body, with the skeletal muscle given the highest priority. Following many months of vigorous exercise stress, the cardiovascular system demonstrates many and significant physiological adaptations which are related to its function of oxygen transport as well as efficient removal of waste products from the muscle cell (9).

It was recognized as early as 1884 that the level of physical work required by the mode of living in various animal species was reflected in autopsy by heart size (4). Since then, x-ray estimations of changes in heart size related to physical activity have confirmed this relationship (27). Athletes participating in the most vigorous endurance type of training demonstrate the largest hearts in proportion to their total body weight. Saltin et al. (28) demonstrated that as little as twenty-one days of physical inactivity (bed rest) results in as much as a 10 percent reduction in heart volume.

Animal experiments have demonstrated an increase in the capillarization (vascularization) of the heart as a result of training (37). Such changes in the blood flow to the heart muscle as a result of training have very important implications for the possible role of exercise in the prevention of heart disease and the rehabilitation of the postcoronary patient (33). If endurance training results in the development of collateral or new blood vessels in the coronary-prone or post-coronary individual then such training may represent the most significant form of prevention and therapy for this major chronic disease entity (8). More longitudinal research is required in this area.

With prolonged training there is an increased ability of the heart to pump blood with each systole or contraction. This is reflected in a higher maximum cardiac output (volume of blood pumped by the heart in one minute) and is due presumably to the increased efficiency of the heart muscle (myocardium) during each contraction or systole, as well as an increase in total blood volume with training, thereby enhancing venous return (21, 2).

It is generally conceded that the trained person has lower resting, working and recovery (postexercise) heart rates. Hoogerwerf (17) found an average heart rate of 50 among participants in the 1928 Amsterdam Olympics. Many of the endurance Olympians had pulse rates of 40, and some even 30, per minute. Ackerman (1) reported significant reductions in heart rate for first year and experienced oarsmen during a season of training. The largest reductions transpired in those athletes who demonstrated the largest increases in heart volume.

There are only limited data regarding the effects of exercise training on the blood pressure. Ekblom et al. (10) concluded that normal persons (not suffering from hypertension or chronic high blood pressure) could expect only small decreases in systolic blood pressure with training. Michael and Gallon (22) demonstrated a significant decrease in systolic blood pressure in an athletic population (college basketball players) with sixteen weeks of training. These positive modifications in blood pressure were reversed after just six weeks of detraining. Boyer and Kasch (5) trained male patients with hypertension for six months in a general fitness program and reported a 12mm Hg decrease in systolic blood pressure.

Schwartz (31) has reported that conditioned subjects show a more qualitative response to gravity stress on the circulatory system (tilt board testing) than sedentary subjects. Subjects exposed to deconditioning through the medium of extended bed rest also experience a depression of qualitative circulatory response to tilt board stress (28, 34). These limited studies suggest that physical conditioning may help to maintain the automatic control of the circulatory system through improved constriction and relaxation of the smooth muscle wall of the vessels.

*Metabolic Adaptations.*  One of the most dramatic physiologic improvements to come with training is that in the area of aerobic power or maximum oxygen consumption. This function may be measured in the human organism at rest or during exercise by obtaining and analyzing an expired air sample and comparing its percent $O_2$ and $CO_2$ with that of the atmospheric air. Knowing the minute pulmonary ventilation, it is then possible to calculate the amount of $O_2$ (liters per minute) utilized to support all of the energetic or metabolic needs of the body tissues during rest or activity. The highest $O_2$ consumption measured in an individual during maximum level work is referred to as the maximum $O_2$ consumption. The physiological mechanisms responsible for delivering large quantities of $O_2$ to the body tissues at rest and work are referred to collectively as the $O_2$ transport system.

The oxygen transport system involves primarily the efficient function of the pulmonary and cardiovascular systems along with efficient extraction or absorption of the oxygen by the muscle cells. Astrand (2) reports from his review of the literature that prolonged endurance training will increase the maximum oxygen consumption from 7 to 19 percent, depending on the duration and intensity of the training program. During detraining imposed by extended bed rest the maximum oxygen consumption can be reduced anywhere from 17 to 31 percent in several weeks (28, 36).

Normally, the metabolic processes in the muscle cell which supply the chemical energy for contraction occur in the presence of $O_2$ and involve the oxidation of glucose. This metabolic utilization of $O_2$ constitutes the *aerobic* source of energy for muscular work. When the $O_2$ transport system does not provide oxygen at a fast enough rate glucose can continue to be metabolized and energy provided without the presence of $O_2$, and this is referred to as the *anerobic* source of energy (or $O_2$ debt). When working anaerobically an intermediate chemical pathway called the lactic acid pathway is utilized. Measurement of lactic acid concentrations in the blood during or after exercise is one means of indirectly determining the level of anaerobic work. Virtually any vigorous physical activity induces both the aerobic and anaerobic metabolic pathways, although the first of these is far more important with respect to the total proportion of energy provided for the support of sustained muscular work.

Several studies support the contention that blood lactate is generally lower during submaximal work following training (10). This condition probably reflects a slower lag time in the response of the aerobic metabolic processes at the beginning of exercise and therefore less reliance upon anaerobic sources. However, during performance of maximum work capacity tests the trained individual demonstrates a higher maximum blood lactate concentration and a lower blood pH than an untrained individual (2). This suggests a greater anaerobic capacity during the latter stages of work as the subject approaches physiological fatigue.

Hollmann (15) has presented data demonstrating that regular endurance training can positively modify the normal decrease in aerobic capacity that occurs with aging. In following sedentary males for twelve to fifteen years they showed an average decline in maximum oxygen consumption of 30 percent. In a similar age group of subjects who remained physically active (endurance activities at least twice per week) during the same period only a 10 percent decline in maximum oxygen consumption occurred. This difference has significant implications regarding aging and exercise tolerance.

Following the cessation of exercise any lactic acid remaining in the blood from anerobic sources of metabolic energy must be resynthesized or oxidized. This removal of lactate from the blood and other body fluids requires oxygen and accounts for the continued elevation of heart rate, blood pressure and pulmonary ventilation after exercise. The whole oxygen transport mechanism must continue to function at higher than base level for several minutes or even hours after exercise, depending upon the intensity and duration of the activity stress. When we measure post-exercise oxygen consumption and compute its elevation above the normal resting or basal level we have estimated the oxygen debt. Oxygen debt is the excess of $O_2$ required to resynthesize or oxidize lactic acid and that $O_2$ necessary to support the continued high level of pulmonary, cardiovascular and metabolic function during recovery from exercise. Robinson's (26) data support the thesis that in the normal, relatively sedentary adult $O_2$ debt decreases with age, along with maximum oxygen consumption.

The effects of training on the maximum $O_2$ debt are not clear, except that the measure can be used to differentiate among sedentary and very active persons. Trained individuals consistently demonstrate an ability to achieve a higher $O_2$ debt. Athletes engaged in short exhaustive kinds of performance such as the 400-meter run demonstrate the highest oxygen debts (14). Astrand (2) reports maximum oxygen debts in excess of 20 liters for an all-out muscular effort of a few minutes duration. The capacity of the trained person to sustain a higher $O_2$ debt probably reflects an increased capacity of the blood to buffer the high concentrations of lactate. When training stops there is a marked drop in postexercise blood lactate concentration (14). Therefore, the endurance trained individual has a significantly higher metabolic reserve than the sedentary person.

*Neuroendocrine Adaptations.* It is now recognized that the so-called training effects of a progressive intensity program, which are recognized by specific physiological changes, are directly related to adaptations in the internal glands of secretion and the autonomic nervous system (that part of the nervous system which regulates organ function and the constancy of the internal environment). Generally, these changes are characterized by modification of adrenal-corticoid function and increased parasympathetic nervous function and sympathetic nervous depression.

Michael (23) summarizes the major neuro-humoral changes associated with long-term physical activity programs and theorizes that certain of them may be related to the organism's increased adaptability to physical or psychic stress. The hormonal alterations involve an increased sensitivity reaction to stress on the part of the adrenal glands' production of epinephrine (adrenaline). Thus, the trained individual may actually be sublimating the physiological manifestation of psychological stress through the medium of exercise.

Increased adrenal function with training is observed in animals by a significant hypertrophy of the gland (3, 18). Various reports are published regarding the acute effects of exercise on the blood and urinary levels of the various adrenal cortical hormones, but generally they appear to increase (32). Very heavy, exhausting levels of work produce as much as a 50 percent increase in the excretion of adrenaline and noradrenaline.

There is other evidence of hormonal involvement in exercise stress. There is a small but significant decrease in blood thyroxin levels in high-level muscular activity, probably caused by increased cellular utilization (7). Ingel and Li (19) used specific pituitary extracts (vasopressin) to induce significant increases in the maximum work capacity of rats.

With respect to autonomic nervous system modification, probably both parasympathetic and sympathetic alterations occur during the course of a long-term training program. The most important modifications, however, probably relate to the parasympathetic function (23). The training modifications of parasympathetic activity are, for example, reflected in lower resting, working and recovery heart rates. Such cardiac adaptation is often referred to as increased vagal tonus (from the vagus nerve, a parasympathetic nerve which moderates heart function).

## SUMMARY

Muscular activity promotes both acute (regulatory) and chronic adaptations in physiological function. These regulatory modifications and adaptations to exercise stress are manifested in pulmonary, cardiovascular, metabolic and endocrine-neural changes. In accordance with the concept of specificity these biological adaptations to exercise stress are highly specialized and require the appropriate training stimulus to be manifested. The specific training regimens for bringing about these various biological adaptations are discussed in Part 4 of this book. Many other qualitative physiological changes have been attributed to regular participation in physical activity, among them increased resistance to communicable diseases, amelioration of the degenerative aspects of the aging process, and improved intellectual function. Such nonspecific effects have not yet been adequately studied and, therefore, valid generalizations regarding relationships to exercise stress would appear unwarranted.

## REFERENCES

1. Ackerman, R. *Zeitachr. f. Klin. Med.* 106 (1927):244.

2. Astrand, P. O. *Textbook of Work Physiology.* New York: McGraw-Hill, 1970.

3. Atwell, W. J. "Effects of Administering Adrenotropic Extract to Hypophysectomized and Thyroidectomized Tadpoles." *American Journal of Physiology* 118 (1937):452.

4. Bergmann, J. "Cher die Grosse des Herzens bei Menschen und Tieren." *Inaug. Dis.* t'niv Munchen. Munich: Wolf und Sohn, 1884.

5. Boyer, J. L., and Kasch, F. W. "Exercise Therapy in Hypertensive Men." *Journal of the American Medical Association* 211 (1970):1668.

6. Consolazio, C. Frank; Johnson, R. E.; Pecora, L. *Physiological Measurements of Metabolic Functions in Man.* New York: McGraw-Hill, 1963.

7. De Nayer, P.; Malvaux, P.; and Ostyn, M. et al. "Serum Free Thyroxin and Binding-Proteins After Muscular Exercise." *Journal of Clinical Endocrinology* 28 (1968):714.

8. Eckstein, R. W. "Effects of Exercise on Coronary Artery Narrowing and Coronary Collateral Circulation." *Circulation Research* 5 (1957):230.

9. Ekblom, B. "Effect of Physical Training on Oxygen Transport System In Man." *Acta Physiolog. Scand.* 51 Suppl. (1969):328.

10. Ekblom, B.; Astrand, P. O.; Saltin, B.; Stenberg, J.; and Wallstrom, B. "Effect of Training on Circulatory Response to Exercise," *Journal of Applied Physiology* 24 (1968):518.

11. Gemmill, C.; Booth, W.; Detrick, J.; and Schiebel, H. *American Journal of Physiology* 96 (1930):265.

12. Gordon, B.; Levine, S. A.; and Wilmaers, A. "Observations on a Group of Marathon Runners." *Archives of Internal Medicine* 33 (1924):425.

13. Guyton, Arthur C. *Textbook of Medical Physiology.* Philadelphia: W. B. Saunders Co., 1969.

14. Hermansen, Lars. "Anerobic Energy Release." *Journal of Medicine and Science in Sports* 1 (March 1969):32.

15. Hollmann, W. *Hochst-und Dauerleistungfahigkeit des Sportlers.* Munich: Johann Ambrosium Barth, 1963.

16. Holmes, E. L. "Pulmonary Function in the Normal Male." *Journal of Applied Physiology* 14 (1959):493.

17. Hoogerwerf, S. "Electrokardiographische Untersuchungen der Amsterdamer Olympiakampfer," *Arbeitsphysiol.* 2 (1929):61.

18. Ingle, D. J. "The Time for the Occurence of Cortico-Adrenal Hypertrophy in Rats During Continued Work." *American Journal of Physiology* 124 (1938):627.

19. Ingle, D. J., and Li, C. H. "Effect of Pituitary Extracts upon the Work Performance of Adrenalectomized-Hypophysectomized Rats, Identification of Vasopressin as a Principle Affecting Work." *Endocrinology* 57 (1955):383.

20. Keele, C., and Niel, E. *Samson Wright's Applied Physiology.* London: Oxford University Press, 1966.

21. Lundhard, J. *Pflugers Arch.* 161 (1915):233.

22. Michael, E. D., and Gallon, A. "Pulse Wave and Blood Pressure Changes Occurring During a Physical Training Program." *Research Quarterly* 31 (March 1960):43.

23. Michael, Ernest D. "Stress Adaptation Through Exercise." *Research Quarterly* 28 (March 1957):50.

24. Mostyn, E. M.; Helle, S.; Gee, J. B. L.; Bentivaglio, L. G.; and Bates, D. V. "Pulmonary Diffusing Capacity of Athletes." *Journal of Applied Physiology* 18 (1963): 687.

25. Newman, F.; Smalley, B. F.; and Thomson, M. L. "Effects of Exercise, Body and Lung Size on C. O. Diffusion in Athletes and Non-Athletes," *Journal of Applied Physiology* 18 (1963):687–95.

26. Robinson, S. "Experimental Studies in Physical Fitness in Relation to Age." *Arbeitsphysiologie* 10 (1938):251.

27. Roskamm, H. "Optimum Patterns of Exercise for the Healthy Adult." *Canadian Medical Association Journal* 22 (1967):895.

28. Saltin, B.; Blomquist, B.; Mitchell, J. H.; Johnson, R. L.; Wildenthal, K.; and Chapman, C. B. "Response to Sub-maximal and Maximal Exercise After Bed Rest and Training." *Circulation* 38, Suppl. 7 (1968).

29. Saltin, B., and Astrand, P. O. "Maximal Oxygen Uptake in Athletes." *Journal of Applied Physiology* 23 (1967):353.

30. Schneider, E. C., and Ring, G. C. "The Influence of a Moderate Amount of Physical Training on the Respiratory Exchange in Breathing During Physical Exercise." *American Journal of Physiology* 91 (1929):103.

31. Schwartz, Esar. "Effect of Gymnastic Training on Orthostatic Efficiency." *Research Quarterly* 39 (May 1968):351.

32. Simonson, Ernst. "Depletion of Adrenal and Other Hormones." In *Physiology of Work Capacity and Fatigue*, edited by E. Simonson. Springfield, Ill.: Charles C Thomas, 1971.

33. South Carolina Heart Association. "Proceedings, National Conference, Exercise in the Prevention, Evaluation, and in the Treatment of Heart Disease." *Journal of the South Carolina Medical Association* 65, Suppl. 1 to no. 12 (December 1969):1.

34. Stevens, P. M.; Miller, P. B.; Lynch, T. N.; Gilbert, C. A.; Johnson, R. L.; and Lamb, L. E. "Effects of Lower Body Negative Pressure on Physiologic Changes Due to Four Weeks of Hypoxic Bed Rest." *Aerospace Medicine* 37 (1966):466.

35. Stuart, D. G., and Collings, W. D. "Comparison of Vital Capacity and Maximum Breathing Capacity of Athletes and Non-Athletes." *Journal of Applied Physiology* 14 (1959):507.

36. Taylor, H. L.; Henschel, A.; Brozek, J.; and Keys, A. "Effects of Bed Rest on Cardiovascular Function and Work Performance." *Journal of Applied Physiology* 2 (1949):223.

37. Vannoti, A., and Pfister, H. "Untersuchungen Zum Studium des Trouniertseins." *Arbeitsphysiol.* 7 (1934):615.

38. West, H. "Clinical Studies on the Respiration VI, A Comparison of Various Standards for the Normal Vital Capacity of the Lungs." *Archives of Internal Medicine* 25 (1920):306.

# PART 4

## Biologic Applications
## of Muscular Activity

**OVERVIEW**   Muscular strength, connective tissue flexibility (joint range of motion) and cardiorespiratory endurance can be significantly altered through the use of an appropriate long-range training program. Efficient strength development is dependent upon the application of a carefully graded progressive-intensity training program. Either isometric or isotonic strength training methods may be implemented. A diverse stretching routine should be incorporated into a balanced fitness program to assist in improvement of postural mechanics and minimize connnective tissue injury. The most careful training design is required for the development and maintenance of the endurance component of physical fitness. The endurance trained individual demonstrates improved biological efficiency and greater physiological reserve capacity during and following exercise stress.

# 8 | Biologic Bases of Strength Development

OBJECTIVES FOR the improvement of strength have been traditionally associated with physical fitness and physical education programs. One reason for this is that the early formal school programs in several parts of this country were associated with the German Turner Gymnastic movement in which performance required high levels of strength. Also, strength has been an important objective in conditioning programs. The changes which take place are gross, measurable and observable. In other words the average individual usually experiences great satisfaction from the increase in strength which occurs as the result of a training program in which he can both feel and see the difference in his muscles in a relatively short period of time. Most of the changes in flexibility and endurance which occur as the result of a conditioning program are not as gross and generally require much longer periods of training to bring about dramatic improvement.

Another reason why strength is so important to any comprehensive fitness program is its relationship to body posture. Usually significant changes in the strength levels of major muscle groups are required to significantly modify any postural malalignment. Much research has been conducted in recent years regarding the physiological phenomena associated with strength development. Two laboratory methods for assessing human strength are depicted in Figures 8.1 and 8.2. Research advances have provided many practical implications for the student interested in developing the most efficient strength training program.

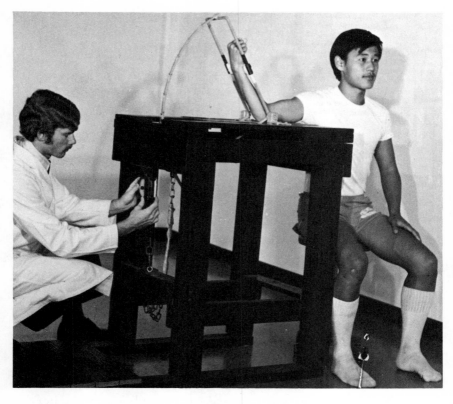

*FIGURE 8.1    Strength Testing, Arm Quadrant.*

### DEFINITION OF STRENGTH

Technically, the strength of a muscle or a muscle group is defined as the force which can be produced through one maximum contraction or collective shortening of the muscle fibers. Practically speaking, however, this is not a very functional definition of strength because most dimensions of human performance require the muscles to function in some kind of repetitive fashion. The most important concept to be derived from the definition, however, is that the more repetitions (contractions) involved in an activity the lower the resistance (in lbs. for example) against which the muscle can effectively work. So as the individual increases the number of times that he repeatedly moves a weight in space, the lower that weight or resistance must be. Because of this, most strength training

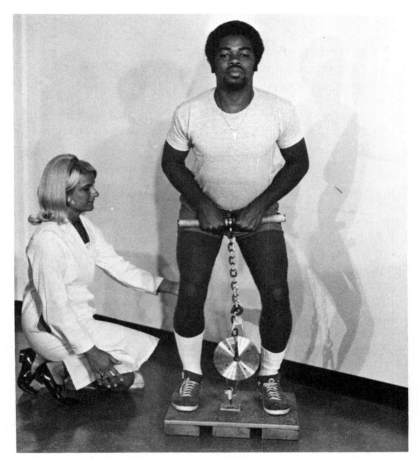

*FIGURE 8.2    Isometric Testing, Leg Dynamometer*

programs involve the use of anywhere from four to fifteen repetitions, depending upon the ultimate level of strength desired. Any significant increase in repetitions much beyond fifteen necessarily involves a significant decrease in the maximum resistance utilized, and thus at some point the subject is developing more muscular endurance than strength (3).

    Logan and Foreman (15) have postulated a strength endurance continuum or spectrum which is represented by maximum strength at one end and maximum endurance at the other. With such a model maximum strength would be represented by one repetition with the maximum resistance. Maximum endurance would be represented by minimum resistance (approximately two-thirds of the maximum or less) and theoretically by maximum repetitions which would vary considerably. In practice most fitness training programs which include weight training place much greater emphasis upon the muscular strength rather than the muscular endurance objective. It appears, however, that a training program which utilizes a resistance level which permits repetitions of approximately ten will result in significant improvement in both muscular strength and endurance (23).

### STRUCTURE OF MUSCLE TISSUE

Strictly from a biological point of view man should be very concerned with his skeletal muscles because they represent most of the tissue volume of the human body. This is indicative of man's inherent capacity and indeed need for movement, and to this extent we are what we are because of our finely integrated neuromuscular system. Skeletal muscle is anatomically classified as connective tissue since it serves the important function of connecting various parts of the skeleton and providing through contraction the capacity for segmental movement.

Microscopically muscles are shown to be composed of long fibers or cells which display a characteristic cross striation, thus often being referred to as striated muscle. Studies with the electron microscope show the striations of skeletal muscle which have been identified as protein bands of differentially refractive material (actin plus myosin). These two bands form the smallest contractile unit of muscle and during contraction the actin filaments slide over the top of the protein filaments, the collective result of which is overall shortening of the muscle. This whole shortening process, however, is dependent upon the continued splitting of Adenosine Triphosphate (ATP) into Adenosine Diphosphate (ADP) and Phosphate (P) along with the oxidation of glucose by the muscle cell (18).

Each muscle fiber is surrounded by a connective, fascial sheath which is attached to the sheaths of other fibers. These fiber sheaths are an outgrowth of larger sheaths which enclose many muscle fibers and thus aid in the collective contraction of many fibers or even an entire muscle. Because each muscle fiber represents a single cell it must have a discrete nerve supply. However, one nerve cell (neuron) may innervate more than one muscle fiber. Generally, the muscles which are involved in very precise and highly coordinated types of movement patterns (as, for example, in the fingers) have a very high nerve supply as contrasted with muscles primarily responsible for very gross movement.

## ENERGY FOR CONTRACTION

The nature of the work or energy requirements for participation in strength types of activity requires the metabolic use of what is referred to in exercise physiology as "aerobic processes." These are the chemical processes by which the body carbohydrate fuels (glucose) are metabolized through the presence of oxygen to produce chemical heat energy in sup-. port of continued muscle contraction. During low levels of activity the lungs and cardiovascular systems supply oxygen to the working muscle cells at a fast enough rate to support metabolization of the carbohydrate foodstuffs and resynthesis of ATP. When, however, the rate and duration of work is increased significantly the respiratory supply of oxygen may be insufficient to support the metabolic energy requirements. In this case new chemical pathways (anerobic processes) are brought into play. The anerobic processes are important during very high level repetitive strength contractions, and during prolonged static contractions in which the muscle blood flow is impeded.

## RESPONSE OF MUSCLE TISSUE TO OVERLOAD

When an individual progressively and systematically increases the load or resistance (overload) which he imposes on a muscle certain predictable biological changes will occur (8). One change which occurs is known as an increase in muscle tonus or tonicity. This is the feeling of firmness or tension within a muscle or group of muscles. It is brought about by an increase in the frequency of the nervous stimuli which cause muscle tissue to contract. Tonus is important in the antigravity muscles of the trunk and legs in maintaining good posture. The abdominal muscles must, for example, maintain a minimum level of strength and tonus in order for the pelvis and abdominal viscera to retain good mechanical position. Round shoulders are similarly related to insufficient strength and tonus in the muscles of the upper back. Thus, the intelligent planning of a strength development program can help to significantly improve posture and body mechanics.

Another change which occurs after long-term participation in a strength training program is an increase in muscle mass or bulk (7). In physiological terms we say that the individual muscle fibers have undergone hypertrophy or increased in their cross-sectional diameter. This phenomenon was first demonstrated experimentally in animals by Siebert (22) in 1928. Such hypertrophy apparently involves no change in muscle cell length but cellular constituents such as the sarcoplasm do increase in volume. There is no conclusive evidence that human beings develop any new muscles or muscle fibers; it is only that each muscle fiber has increased its microscopic diameter. Results from recent animal experiments, however, have shown that long-term overload training may create some new muscle fibers, although this represents only a minor proportion of the total increase in muscle volume (13, 21).

It is because of hypertrophy response that strength training can be used to change bodily proportions. By stressing certain muscle groups and not others in weight training programs it is possible to affect muscle bulk and tonus on a differential basis. This process effectively modifies the soft tissue proportions of the different body parts. This result is possible, given enough time and a training stimulus of sufficiently high intensity, only because the neuromuscular system is so biologically adaptive.

The physiological opposite of hypertrophy is known as atrophy and is characterized by a wasting of muscle tissue (10). It is observed in persons who are bedridden for long periods, or who have a limb immobilized in a splint or cast. Muscle atrophy is also often observed in persons who have allowed themselves to become very sedentary, particularly in middle and old age.

Since muscle which is increasingly stressed or overloaded responds biologically by increasing in size it is not surprising that there is a high correlation between muscle girth (cross-sectional diameter) and muscle strength (11). The amount of increase in strength and hypertrophy, however, is directly proportional to the amount of overload (or increase in the intensity of the training stimulus—the resistance factor)(12). It should also be recognized that there are great individual differences in potential for both maximum strength improvement and the biological adaptation of hypertrophy. To what extent the differences are explainable on a genetic basis is not clear at the present time. Since there are tremendous motivational variables involved in the perserverance required for participation in a longitudinal strength training program, it may well be that some of the differences can be explained on a psychological basis.

In general, there are rather significant differences in strength performances between the male and female. At any time after seven years of age the average female's maximum strength performance is roughly 60 percent of the male and 80 percent when the data are corrected for difference in body size (1). To what extent this differential response is purely physiological rather than a culturally learned pattern of behavior is hypothetical. It seems reasonable to assume that in the American culture the feminine ideal is such that high levels of muscular strength development are not particularly desirable. Research by Rodahl (20) suggests that the potential for strength and therefore hypertrophy development is partly a function of the testosterone or male sex hormones. This lesser hypertrophy response on the part of the female could be a distinct advantage since it might permit her to use weight training for improvement of body mechanics and muscle tonus without running the risk of developing muscles which are too big or unfeminine. It should be well understood, however, that there are great individual differences within both sexes with respect to strength and hypertrophy response.

### SPECIFICITY OF STRENGTH

Strength, not unlike the phenomenon of flexibility, is highly specific. Therefore, the manner or conditions under which training occurs for the improvement of strength determines to a great extent what kind of strength we develop. There are various ways in which muscles can contract or be overloaded. Each of these are dealt with briefly below.

*Isotonic vs. Isometric Contraction.* Recently, much has been written in the scientific and popular literature regarding isometric training techniques for the improvement of human strength. This method of training varies significantly from traditional techniques utilizing barbells and dumbbells. Essentially, isometric contraction may be thought of as a static contraction (relatively speaking there is little or no movement of the joint) whereas isotonic contraction usually involves the complete excursion of joint movement. The advantages and disadvantages of isometric training techniques for the purpose of improving the strength component of physical fitness have been debated for years. The important concept to understand here is that the kind of strength which is developed with isotonic training (sometimes referred to as dynamic strength) is quite different from that developed in an isometric program. Laboratory techniques have been developed for measuring the force developed by a muscle group while contracting isometrically or isotonically and although the correlation is high ($r = .8$) electromyographic studies indicate that very different neural patterns are involved (9).

It is well recognized that when an individual increases his strength 25 percent in eight weeks, part of this is a result of adaptation at the muscle level (i.e., fiber enlargement) and part is a result of neurological adaptation. Thus we may think of improvement in strength as being partly a learned phenomenon and when a person "learns" to contract his muscles isotonically and exert greater force, he has not necessarily "learned" to accomplish this to the same degree isometrically. Isotonic training techniques are generally considered to be more appropriate for purposes of strength improvement as part of a physical fitness program. One chief advantage is that the individual can see and measure his progress. In addition, it is assumed that since man uses his muscular strength in everyday activities in a dynamic fashion, that strength which is developed isotonically is more functional and practicable than that developed isometrically.

*Concentric vs. Eccentric Contraction.* When consideration is given to the manner in which a muscle contracts isotonically it becomes apparent that this can occur in two different ways. The most common is referred to as concentric contraction, since the muscle fibers shorten as the muscle develops greater tension and exerts more force. This method of shortening contraction is the manner in which one normally trains with weights for improving isotonic strength. It should be recognized, however, that occasionally one may develop high levels of tension in a muscle and gradually let go or reduce that tension as the muscle fibers lengthen. A good example of this is the lowering of a heavy weight from shoulder height to the ground. In such an instance the weight is grasped, developing maximum tension, and then the tension is reduced carefully as the muscle lengthens. This is referred to as lengthening or eccentric contraction. As the reader would suspect, laboratory investigations have demonstrated that strength developed with eccentric methods of contraction is quite specific and different than concentric strength.

*Effect of Range of Motion.* When discussing the specificity of strength it is also important to understand the implications of training at various degrees in the range of joint motion (14). Whether an individual utilizes isometric or isotonic training methods he will tend to gain optimum strength improvement at those angles at which he trains or develops tension in the muscle. Thus, an individual who trains isometrically only with his arm in a completely extended position will become quite strong in that particular anatomical position but will increase his strength very little at other positions. Or, the individual who isotonically overloads the biceps muscles by doing arm curls through one half of the range of arm flexion will not get very strong beyond that range. Or, another way to say it is that he will get stronger biceps for doing one-half arm curls but not much stronger for doing full arm curls.

Muscle strength is a very complicated function. It involves many physiological as well as psychological variables. An understanding of the basic training principles which will lead to the most efficient development of strength is necessary for the individual interested in planning a long-term balanced program which will significantly improve posture, body mechanics and contribute to the overall objectives of physical fitness.

Elementary principles of safety and training techniques are discussed below for both isometric and isotonic programs.

### ISOMETRICS

As mentioned previously, isometric training methods involve static contractions of the muscles without joint movement. Several isometric training techniques are shown in Figures 8.3, 8.4 and 8.5. Such routines can be designed for any major muscle groups of the body utilizing the floor, a chair, wall or a doorway for resistive purposes. In fact, the major advantages of isometric strength training are that no special equipment or facilities are required and very little time is required for executing the movements. Therefore, an individual can develop and maintain good muscle tonus with just several minutes of exercise per day. The research of Muller and Rohmert (17) demonstrates that the isometric contractions should be held for at least five or six seconds and repeated several times daily with optimum results obtained with about ten contractions. Training sessions should be conducted no fewer than three or four times weekly. For the first several weeks of such a training program the individual should consciously avoid maximum contractions, and work at approximately two-thirds tension or resistance in the muscles.

Over a period of several weeks, as the muscle and other connective tissue adjusts to the imposed isometric strain the subject can gradually increase the level of tension and eventually work at maximum resistance which will bring about the greatest increase in strength (maximum gains of 5 percent weekly), tonus and hypertrophy. With such a graded progressive training program, muscle soreness and connective tissue injury can be minimized. During held isometric contractions continuous breath holding should be avoided since this may impair normal circulation. Therefore, normal cyclic breathing is to be encouraged during isometric muscle contraction. Also, in accordance with earlier statements regarding the specificity of strength and joint angle, it is advisable to isometrically train the muscles of the arm and legs at several angles. In this way the individual "learns" to be strong at various points in the full range of motion and the strength developed will presumably have more carry-over to his performance in everyday situations. He should recognize that after several months of participation in an isometric strength program it is difficult to maintain his motivation for maximum contraction. One reason for this is that he has no practical feedback, or measure of performance. For this reason many persons interested in long-range reconditioning or fitness programs use isometric techniques as a lead-up activity prior to initiation

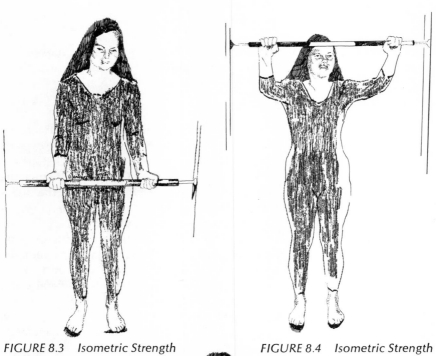

FIGURE 8.3    Isometric Strength
Training

FIGURE 8.4    Isometric Strength
Training

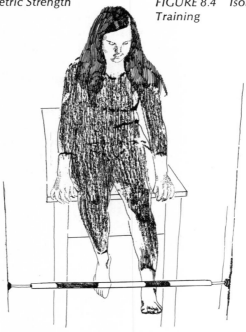

FIGURE 8.5    Isometric Strength
Training

of an isotonic strength program. It also should be noted that isometrics, unlike isotonic training programs, provide only a minimal stimulus for muscle hypertrophy (19), improved cardiovascular function (16), and muscular endurance (6).

### ISOTONICS

As emphasized earlier in this chapter, resistive exercises which involve full excursion of the body joints are most commonly used for strength improvement as part of a body conditioning or fitness program. This may be accomplished by working with a partner as depicted in Figures 8.6 and 8.7, or with dumbells, barbells, or leg weights.

The use of resistance provided by a partner offers a convenient and quick method for improving isotonic strength. Such a partner should be

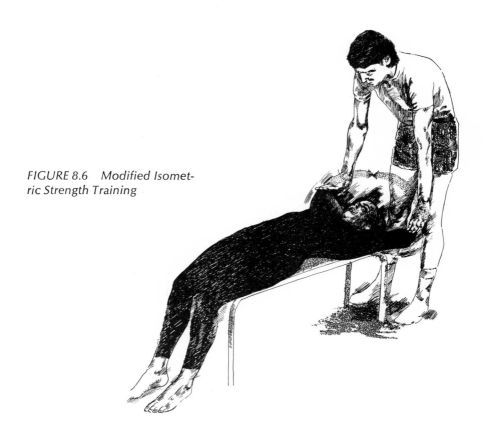

FIGURE 8.6 Modified Isometric Strength Training

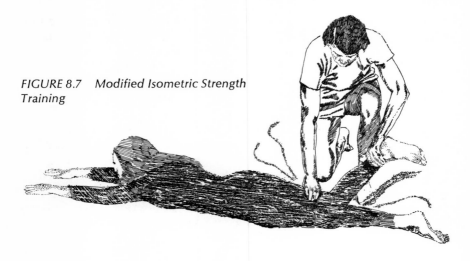

*FIGURE 8.7    Modified Isometric Strength Training*

of approximately the same body size and strength level. Otherwise it will be necessary for the stronger partner to exercise considerable restraint while providing resistance for the weaker partner. The body part being resisted should be allowed to travel through the complete range of motion with lesser resistance being provided at the beginning and end of the movement. This is because one generally tends to be strongest in the most often used middle range of motion, and correspondingly weaker at the extreme ranges of motion. In initiating such an isotonic training program with a partner providing resistance it is best to begin with minimum resistance and over a period of several weeks work towards maximum levels of muscular contraction. There is considerable learning required on the part of the resisting partner since different body parts vary in strength and even different muscles in the same body part will vary in strength potential. By learning to analyze the role of the many muscle groups, routines can be developed so as to provide a balanced strength improvement program.

The use of weights such as barbells or dumbbells is undoubtedly the most reliable method of improving strength since one's progress is constantly being measured. Typical isotonic routines are outlined in Figures 8.8 through 8.15. There are many programs which have been developed for optimum strength performance and the individual may decide for himself which meets his time and overall fitness requirements. One of the earliest isotonic strength programs was developed by de Lorme (4) for therapeutic purposes in the rehabilitation of men who had various kinds

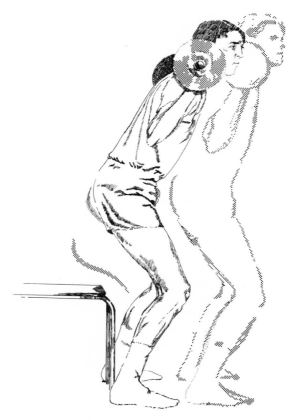

FIGURE 8.8    Isotonic Leg Press

of lower extremity disabilities. The original program has been modified by other clinicians, teachers and researchers for various purposes, but the basic principles underlying the original model are still valid and can be applied to the strength dimension of a physical fitness program.

The de Lorme technique (5) involves initial determination of the maximum resistance or weight which can be moved through the full range of motion ten times. The basal strength level is referred to as repetition maximum (RM). Thereafter, using the progressive resistance principle the subject trains approximately every other day (or 3–4 times per week) using three sets of 10 RM with a brief rest period between each set.

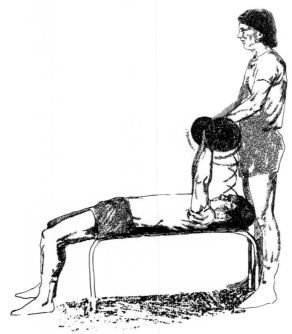

*FIGURE 8.9    Isotonic Bench Press*

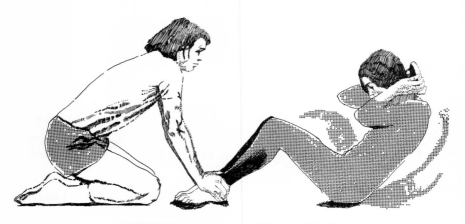

*FIGURE 8.10    Isotonic Abdominal Curl*

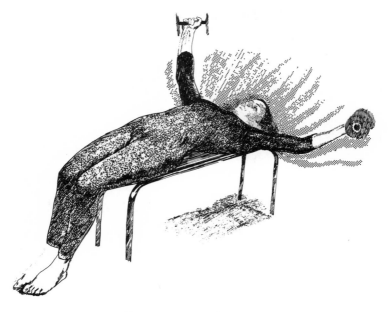

FIGURE 8.11    Isotonic Supine Arm Raise

The following example assumes a 10 RM of 200 lbs:

1st set—10 repetitions at approximately 50% of 10 RM or 100 lbs.
2nd set—10 repetitions at approximately 75% of 10 RM or 150 lbs.
3rd set—10 repetitions of 100% of 10 RM or 200 lbs.

This routine is followed for each isotonic exercise and the baseline 10 RM may be increased approximately 5 percent per week. However, as one approaches his maximum strength potential smaller improvement increments are to be expected. Eventually a plateau or leveling effect is to be expected, after which time it is difficult to maintain the necessary motivation for even small regular improvements in strength.

Certain muscle groups will show very rapid initial gains in strength simply because of their relatively weak condition. The stronger muscle groups which the individual uses in resistive fashion in everyday activities already possess a large percent of their maximum strength potential and will not show such dramatic initial gains. When the plateau effect is observed over a long period of time it may be desirable to decrease the number of repetitions for several training sessions so as to provide the opportunity to increase the resistance factor. After increasing the resist-

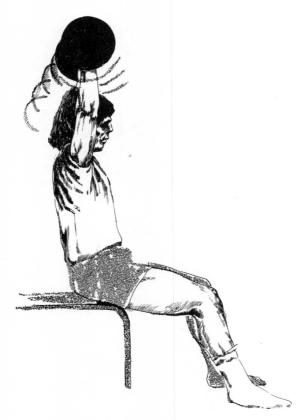

FIGURE 8.12    *Isotonic Military Press*

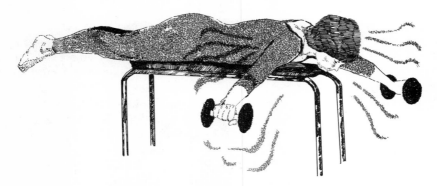

FIGURE 8.13    *Isotonic Prone Arm Raise*

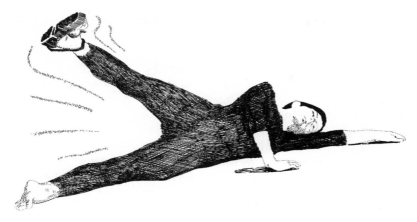

FIGURE 8.14    Isotonic Side Leg Raise

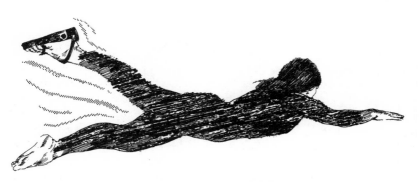

FIGURE 8.15    Isotonic Back Leg Raise

ance factor the subject then progressively increases the number of repetitions until he reaches the maximum again, at which time he may again lower the repetition factor and increase the resistance. Berger and Harris (3) provide for such a variable repetition program and recommend that no fewer than six repetitions and no more than twelve repetitions be utilized.

There is nothing magic about the maximum number of repetitions being established as ten or twelve. As mentioned earlier in the chapter, approximately this number of repetitions appears to be practical because it results in significant improvement in both muscle strength and endurance, and therefore should have maximum carry-over to sports and other performance activities. If the primary objective is upon maximum muscle strength, however, then a program utilizing 4 RM to 8 RM would appear to be more efficient (2). The traditional de Lorme program based on the 10 RM base is apparently more beneficial for the improvement of muscle bulk or hypertrophy (19). That program is to be preferred, then, for the individual interested in using isotonic resistive training to reproportion his body parts by differentially changing muscle mass. For the individual who is interested specifically in increasing the endurance of his muscles, that is, his ability to sustain prolonged stress or effort, then higher repetitions of anywhere from fifteen to thirty repetitions would be desirable. Such high level repetitions would necessarily require a significant reduction in the resistance factor.

### TRAINING GUIDELINES

There are some basic guides to be considered in establishing any kind of progressive resistance strength improvement program. First, a light warm-up session should precede each training session. This warm-up should consist of light calisthenic activities and include static stretching of the major muscle groups so as to minimize the possibility of connective tissue injury. Extreme care should be taken by those persons attempting to recondition themselves after years of muscular inactivity. They should begin their strength development program with very low resistance and only gradually approach, after several weeks, training intensities with maximum muscular tension. Special attention should be given to body posture during performance of resistive routines. Good body mechanics which provide ample stabilization and allow linear stress to be imposed on the connective tissue while muscular contractions occur are to be emphasized. Good stabilization is provided if only the body part performing the resistive exercise is allowed to move, with no other extraneous movement of other body segments. Resistive repetitions should be performed at a moderate rhythmic rate with a short rest period between each set. As emphasized earlier, normal rhythmic breathing is utilized with no breath holding. Attention to these simple principles will allow one to pursue a safe, comfortable, strength improvement program and will contribute most effectively to improvement of muscle tonus, body posture, efficient performance of daily motor requirements, and improvement of general physical fitness.

## SUMMARY

Neuromuscular strength is very important to body posture and maintenance of good biomechanics. The external physical dimensions of the body are primarily determined by the size and tonus of the skeletal muscles. Muscle size and tonus can be increased through progressive overload. By overloading some muscle groups and not others it is possible to selectively reproportion body parts. Insufficient mechanical stress on the neuromuscular system results in a wasting of muscle tissue (atrophy), postural malalignment, and inefficient movement patterns or biomechanics. Sufficient muscular strength is also important for the prevention of connective tissue injury during participation in vigorous recreational and sports activity. Progressive, graded overload should be carefully incorporated into any strength development training program.

## REFERENCES

1. Asmussen, E., as reported by P. O. Astrand in *Textbook of Work Physiology*. New York: McGraw-Hill, 1970, p. 94.

2. Berger, R. A. "Comparison of Static and Dynamic Strength Increases." *Research Quarterly* 33 (1962):329.

3. Berger, R. A., and Harris, M. W. "Effects of Various Repetitive Rates in Weight Training on Improvements in Strength and Endurance." *American Corrective Therapy Journal* 20 (1966):205.

4. DeLorme, T. L. "Restoration of Muscle Power by Heavy Resistance Exercises." *Journal of Bone and Joint Surgery* 37A (1945):645.

5. DeLorme, T. L., and Watkins, A. L. *Progressive Resistance Exercise*. New York: Appleton-Century-Crofts, 1951.

6. Dennison, J. D.; Howell, M. L.; and Morford, W. R. "Effect of Isometric and Isotonic Exercise Programs Upon Muscular Endurance." *Research Quarterly* 32 (1961):348.

7. deVries, H. *Physiology of Exercise for Physical Education and Athletics*. Dubuque, Iowa: Wm. C. Brown Co., 313, 1966.

8. Hellebrandt, F. A., and Houtz, S. J. "Mechanisms of Muscle Training In Man; Experimental Demonstration of the Overload Principle." *Physical Therapy Review* 35 (1968):371–83.

9. Hettinger, T. *Physiology of Strength*. Springfield, Ill.: Charles C Thomas, 1961.

10. Hettinger, T., and Muller-Weeker, H. "Histologische and Chemischz Verand er ungen der Skeletmuskulatur bei Atrophie." *Arbeitsphysioligie*, 15 (1954):459.

11. Ikai, M., and Fukunaga, T. "Calculation of Muscle Strength per Unit Cross Sec-

tional Area of Human Muscle by Means of Ultrasonic Measurement." *Int. Z. angew. Physiol. einschl. Arbeitsphysiol* 26 (1968) :26.

12. Lang, B. *Uber Lunkionelle Anpassury.* Berlin: Springer Verlag, 1919.

13. Linge, B. van. "The Response of Muscle to Strenuous Exercise." *Journal of Bone and Joint Surgery* 44 (1962) :711.

14. Logan, G. A. "Differential Applications of Resistance and Resulting Strength Measured at Varying Degrees of Knee Extension." Ph.D. dissertation, University of Southern California, 1960.

15. Logan, G. A., and Foreman, K. E. "Strength Endurance Continuum." *Physical Educator* 18 (1961) :103.

16. Morehouse, L. E., and Rasch, P. J. *Sports Medicine for Trainers.* Philadelphia: W. B. Saunders Co., 1963.

17. Muller, E. Å., and Rohmert, W. "Die Geschurndigkeit der Muskelkroft Zunahme bei Isometrischen Training." *Int. Z. Angew Physiol einsehl. Arbeitsphysiologie* 19 (1963) :403.

18. Needham, D. M. "Energy Production in Muscle." *British Medical Bulletin* 12 (1956) :194.

19. Rasch, P. J., and Morehouse, L. E. "Effect of Static and Dynamic Exercises on Muscular Strength and Hypertrophy." *Journal of Applied Physiology* 11 (1957) :29.

20. Rodahl, K.; Issekutz, B., Jr.; Blizzard, J. J.; and Demos, C. H. "The Effect of Anti-anabolic Steroids on Muscle Strength, Nitrogen Balance and Body Weight in Healthy Subjects." Unpublished Manuscript, 1965.

21. Reitsma, W. "Regeneratie, Volumetrische en Numerieke Hypertrophie van Skelet-spieren bij Kikkeren Rat." *Acad. Proefschrift, Vrije Universiteit Te Amsterdam,* 1965.

22. Siebert, W. W. "Investigations on Hypertrophy of the Skeletal Muscle." *Zeit-schrift Furr Klinische Madizin* 109 (1928) :350.

23. Yessis, M. "Relationships Between Varying Combinations of Resistances and Repetitions in the Strength-Endurance Continuum." Ph.D. dissertation, University of Southern California, 1963.

# 9 | Biologic Bases of Flexibility Development

FLEXIBILITY MAY be defined in several different ways—as mobilization, freedom to move, or technically as the measurement of range of motion in the body joints. Essentially, it involves the role of several different kinds of connective tissue in limiting the various dimensions of joint motion. It is rather generally assumed by physical educators that flexibility is an important objective of physical fitness (8, 9, 11). Improved flexibility is usually categorized along with strength, cardiorespiratory endurance, and so on, as a suitable objective in conditioning programs. It is of particular importance in reconditioning programs since people who have been inactive for long periods of time usually experience some shortening of joint connective tissue. Gross shortening of connective tissue may result in postural abnormalities with associated pain syndromes as well as increased susceptibility to injury.

Some of the major changes which transpire in skeleton, muscles and connective tissue as a result of muscular activity were outlined in Chapter 6. In order to better understand the relationship between joint range of motion and physical activity it is necessary to better understand the physiological characteristics of the various connective tissues and how they are modified with age, body posture and specialized stress. The latter part of this chapter provides some practical guidelines for the development of a training program to modify connective tissue and improve flexibility.

## CHARACTERISTICS OF CONNECTIVE TISSUE

There are several types of connective tissue which limit the extent of joint motion. The ligaments (bone to bone) are the most important connective tissue of the body and consist primarily of a ground substance (collagen) which is practically inextensible, thus providing great stability to the joints. Since, however, the ligaments are quite inelastic, they are subject to injury (sprain) and require several weeks to form scar tissue and heal. When the major ligaments of a joint are severely damaged then the adjacent muscles must be significantly strengthened (through systematic weight training, for example) in order to provide joint stabilization. Guidelines for the development of strength training programs are outlined in Chapter 8.

Tendons connect muscle tissue to bone and consist primarily of heavy parallel collagenous fibers which form strong narrow bands (for example, the Achilles tendon) or rounded cords. Tendons are described anatomically as having great tensile strength and being practically inelastic. Repeated mechanical stress on ligaments or tendons appears to result in some lengthening of the tissue, but whether the tissue is then weakened (as through stretching) is somewhat controversial (1, 11, 13).

Cartilage tissue is found in various body sites including the interior of the joint proper. A special kind of cartilage, designated hyaline, lines the bony surfaces which are exposed to friction during joint motion, thus acting as a buffer. At this anatomical site the cartilage is very hard and tough and normally does not limit joint flexibility. During the latter stages of exhaustive exercise, however, the joint cartilage may swell and increase in thickness, thus slightly limiting excursion of the joint (7). Also, since the joint hyaline cartilage is exposed to a great frictional component and has no ability to repair itself, it often degenerates following joint trauma and may require surgical excision. A frequent site of such trauma and degeneration is the meniscii cartilages of the knee joint. The joint hyaline cartilage is also a frequent site of excessive mechanical wear and osteoarthritis.

The skeletal muscle fibers are among the most supple and pliable of all the connective tissue. Electron microscope (ultra microphotography) studies have shown that the muscle tissue is richly endowed with an elastin substance which gives it considerable resiliency (12). This elastin component is probably found in the sarcolemma (muscle cell membrane) and the sarcoplasm (muscle cell protoplasm). The connective tissue which forms enveloping sheaths around muscle is known as fascia. It consists principally of collagenous fibrils although the fascia of certain muscles (those most functional in everyday activity) are quite rich in elastin connective material (2). Each individual muscle fiber is surrounded with a thin layer of fascia and each bundle of muscle fibers is also enclosed in this type of connective tissue.

Due to the physiological makeup of the muscle fibers and their fascial covering they are significantly involved in flexibility and apparently do respond to stretching. There is strong clinical opinion that muscle fascia becomes increasingly susceptible to fibrocytic contracture and shortening with age and lack of exercise (9). It is postulated that such shortening of muscle fascia places undue pressure on nerve pathways and muscle tissue, resulting in a host of neuromuscular pain syndromes (3). It has been suggested, therefore, that stretching might serve to alleviate many of the common neuromuscular syndromes of middle-aged or older people.

## SPECIFICITY OF FLEXIBILITY

Although we tend to think of flexibility as related to fitness in very general terms (that is, people are generally very flexible or inflexible in the body joints) research studies do not substantiate this. In fact, there is probably no such phenomenon as general flexibility and further, specific measures of flexibility are only indicative of the range of motion in the specific joints measured and cannot be used to validly predict flexibility in other body parts. In fact, there are usually significant differences in flexibility in the same joints on different sides of the body (8). Thus, the phenomenon of flexibility in different body parts apparently reflects the different stresses and strains which have been imposed on them over long periods of time. This is consonant with the concept of specific biological adaptation as previously discussed in Part 3 of this book.

The specificity concept is important to understand in terms of evaluating the individual's own pattern of flexibility for purposes of fitness. He will probably find that in certain movements of some joints he is exceptionally hyperflexible, whereas in others he is quite inflexible (hypoflexible). These differences reflect genetic variation, personal activity patterns, and the specialized mechanical strains which the individual has imposed on his connective tissue.

It is also important to understand that there is an optimum range of flexibility for each movement of each joint. Certainly the specialized athlete such as a gymnast requires highly specific patterns of flexibility to facilitate certain kinds of performance. But the average young adult who is not participating in highly competitive athletics wishes to achieve a more balanced or optimum range of motion. For purposes of the nonathlete, neither hyperflexibility nor hypoflexibility is desirable since either may predispose towards postural malalignment and connective tissue injury. Therefore, the optimum level of flexibility for any individual is that which facilitates his specialized physical activity performance and minimizes the development of postural deviation and connective tissue injury. The young woman who participates in modern dance activities regularly requires a much different pattern of flexibility in the various joints than the girl who pursues only golf for recreational purposes.

### POSTURE AND FLEXIBILITY

The exact relationship between the development of postural syndromes and range of joint motion is not entirely clear. It is generally accepted clinically by orthopedists and physical medicine specialists, however, the most cases of inflexibility are characterized by shortened connective tissue on one side of the joint and weakened muscles on the other. For example, round shoulders are usually associated with shortening of the muscles and other connective tissue on the front of the shoulder girdle and stretching and weakening of the posterior muscles which normally hold the shoulders back. The condition presumably may be alleviated by stretching the shortened connective tissue and muscles and strengthening the weakened muscles. This lengthening-strenghthening principle may be generally applied in attempting to help alleviate most of the common postural syndromes.

Dysmenorrhea (excessive or painful menstruation) is often clinically described as a postural deviation involving shortening of ligamentous connective tissue around the uterus. Billig (3) recommends a routine which presumably stretches the ligamentous tissue and reportedly assists in ameliorating the condition.

### AGE AND FLEXIBILITY

Many studies have been conducted on the changing flexibility patterns of boys and girls of elementary and secondary school age (7). The findings seem to be somewhat contradictory; however, in general terms the trends with increasing age were negative but slight. Also, girls tended to be slightly more flexible than boys. Very little longitudinal scientific study has been made of changing flexibility patterns in the middle-aged and older populations. It has been clinically demonstrated, however, that human beings tend to become increasingly inflexible with age (5). But whether the shortening of connective tissue is mostly a concommitant of the physiological degenerative processes of aging or whether it simply reflects reduced activity levels is not clear. It may well be that since people become more sedentary as they get older much of their connective tissue adaptively shortens and they become somewhat more inflexible. It would seem logical for middle-aged and older people to place a high priority upon the maintenance of optimum flexibility patterns through the use of regular stretching routines.

The low back pain syndromes, so common in the middle-aged and elderly populations, are often alleviated by stretching of the muscle and muscle fascia (10). It may well be that such syndromes could be avoided in young adulthood by a preventive program which emphasizes functional strengthening and stretching. Special consideration should be given in one's fitness program to mobilization and stretching of the spinal and back extensor muscles and connective tissue. The concepts of flexibility training which are outlined below are designed to serve as practical guide-lines for the development of a program for the general improvement of body flexibility.

### DEVELOPMENT OF FLEXIBILITY

*Linear Stretch.* In order to obtain maximum improvement of flexi-bility and minimize the possibility of injury to the connective tissue the body position should be such that the stretch is applied parallel to the muscle fibers and other connective tissue rather than diagonal to or at an angle to the muscle fibers. The application of this principle can be best understood by analyzing each stretching routine and noting the muscles being stretched. It should be noted that the optimum stretch position in each case is one which produces stretch along the axis of the muscle belly rather than at a diagonal. Thus, it is important in learning each of your stretching routines that you carefully determine the most efficient body position and posture.

*Active Stretch Techniques.* For general purposes of physical fitness, active rather than passive stretching should be utilized. The passive types of stretching which require the use of another person to impose the stretch are used primarily by trained therapists for rehabilitation purposes and can be dangerous when the operator is not highly skilled. Active tech-niques, in which the subject applies the stretch himself and controls the amount of progressive stress imposed on the connective tissue, are pre-ferred for use by laymen. The passive techniques should only be used by professionally trained therapists and are mentioned here only because some popular publications on physical fitness have often advocated their use.

*Static Stretch Techniques.*  There are two general types of active stretching which have been developed by dancers, gymnasts and other performers interested in developing maximum flexibility. The ballistic stretch involves repetitive rebound movements which are aimed toward gradual progressive increase of joint motion, and is sometimes referred to as a fast stretch. This type of stretch places considerable stress on the connective tissue and may even result in trauma. In addition, it induces a neurological reflex (myotatic stretch reflex) which causes contraction of the muscle while the individual is attempting to lengthen or stretch it. Certainly the technique will result in residual muscle and joint pain if it is used by persons who have been sedentary for a long period of time. Because of this its usage is not recommended for inclusion in a fitness program and should only be attempted after the individual has increased his flexibility using static stretching. The static stretch method is recommended for general purposes of a fitness program (6).

The static stretch involves the use of a held stretch position which may or may not be repeated. It is usually described as a controlled or slow stretch. Essentially, the subject attempts to gently and gradually increase the degree of stretch. The static stretch involves no bobbing or jerking movements. If the poorly conditioned person uses only the static stretch method for improving flexibility he will be able to progress more rapidly in his training program.

In order to achieve optimum flexibility results from each stretching routine, the static position should be held for several seconds. During the held stretch you should be conscious of a feeling of increased stretch developing in the muscle and other connective tissues. After several days of repeated stretching you may wish to hold each static position for longer periods of time.

*Increased Repetitions.*  A beginning program of flexibility training might require the performance of each of the routines only once in each training session. However, as the training progresses, an attempt should be made to gradually increase the amount of static stretch imposed on each successive repetition of each routine. If this principle is adhered to very significant gains in range of motion will be observed in just a matter of weeks.

*Pain Limitations.*  Fortunately, it is almost impossible, from a physiological point of view, to seriously injure or damage connective tissue through the use of a carefully developed static stretch program.

Biologically, our connective tissue is well equipped with receptors or sensors which are very sensitive to stretch stimuli. The neurological feedback from these stretch receptors is considerable and helps to keep us aware of the level of stress which is developing. Very high levels of stretch stimulate pain receptors and this becomes then a very limiting factor. An interesting point, however, is that through progressively increased stretching over several weeks, the level at which the pain receptors are stimulated changes, so apparently there is some adaptation which takes place. It should be recognized, however, that in order to significantly improve flexibility the subject must go a *little* beyond the point of pain in each training session.

*Training Sessions.* In order to appreciate the most dramatic improvement in range of motion you should practice the flexibility routines at least three times per week. There is nothing magic about this number but it appears to represent the optimum conditioning stimulus for persons concerned with range of motion for physical fitness. Ideally, of course, the most significant changes could be made in joint flexibility if these routines were practiced each day, particularly at the beginning of a reconditioning program for a person who has been relatively inactive for a long period of time. Stretching should always be included as part of a warm-up routine prior to gross vigorous activity. This will help to reduce the possibility of connective tissue injury.

*Specificity Stretching.* The kinds of flexibility which we develop through certain kinds of training programs are, like most training responses, highly specific from a biological point of view. As pointed out in the first part of this chapter, the performance of different activities requires specialized adaptation on the part of the various connective tissue and results in specialized patterns of joint range of motion. Thus, the gymnast demonstrates a much different pattern of joint flexibility than the ballet dancer, and the football lineman is in certain respects quite flexible, and in other respects quite inflexible. This is indicative of the adaptive changes which our connective tissue undergoes in response to the rather specific kinds of stresses which we impose on it. To understand this is important, since it has been rather well demonstrated that specific stretching should be an important part of the warm-up procedure in order to minimize the possibility of connective tissue injury, particularly in "all out" activities.

The warm-up stretching routine should be as much as possible like the kind of stretch imposed during the performance of the activity, which is to say specific preparation for specific performance. The football lineman has to analyze the body positions he assumes and the limits of motion to which he is normally exposed in order to intelligently plan his warm-up stretch. The modern dancer and the high hurdler have to include some ballistic stretch in their training and warm-up regimen, but only after many months of specifically and progressively working up to this kind of connective tissue stress. Similarly, the swimmer requires a much different kind of stretching warm-up than does the track sprinter or the wrestler.

Which kind of stretching is required for a given performance activity requires a biomechanical and anatomical analysis of the muscles involved. For this purpose the reader is referred to an elementary kinesiology reference (4). The simple static stretch routines outlined below will provide the reader with a regimen designed to stress the major joints and contribute to one's overall physical fitness provided the above guidelines are adhered to. These routines may also be used as part of a general warm-up for participation in calisthenic or other light fitness activities.

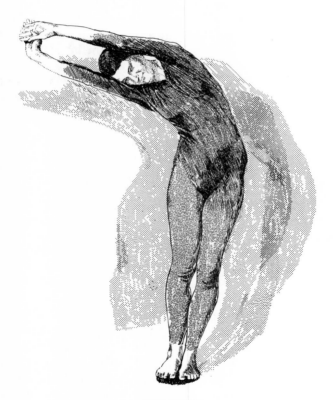

*FIGURE 9.1*

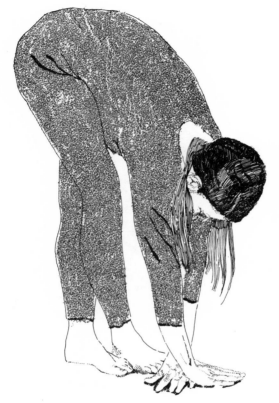

*FIGURE 9.2*

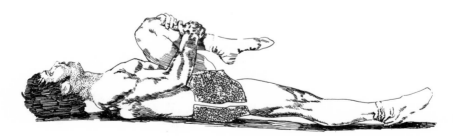

*FIGURE 9.3*

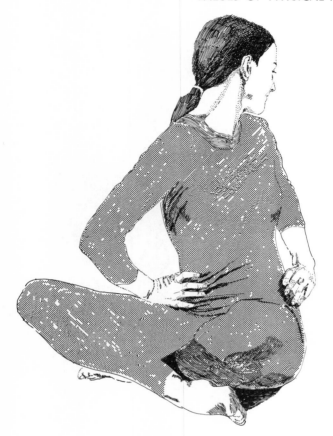

FIGURE 9.4

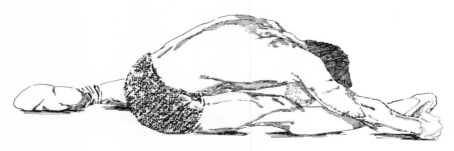

FIGURE 9.5

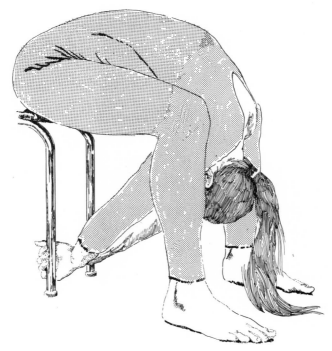

*FIGURE 9.6*

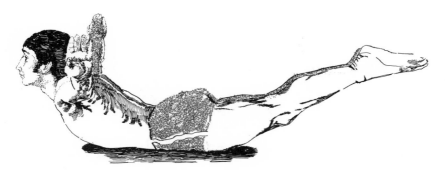

*FIGURE 9.7*

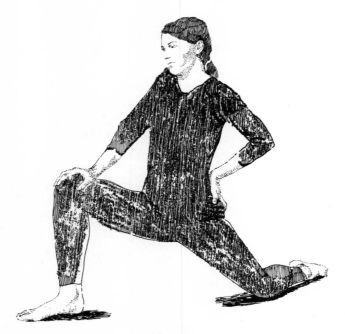

FIGURE 9.8

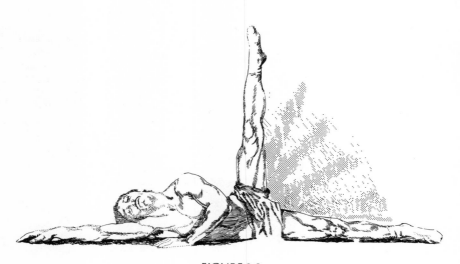

FIGURE 9.9

## SUMMARY

Flexibility or joint range of motion is an important component of a fitness conditioning program. Persons lacking in flexibility suffer from postural deviation, pain from pressure on nerve pathways, and increased susceptibility to connective tissue injury. The connective tissues which limit joint motion are muscle, muscle fascia, tendons, ligaments and cartilage. Flexibility is highly specific, and therefore may vary significantly from one body part to another. Specific active static stretching routines should be utilized to increase joint range of motion. Since it appears that the connective tissue becomes less resilient with increasing age, stretching routines should be a regular and important component of the adult fitness regimen. Stretching should always be included in the warm-up routine prior to participation in vigorous muscular activity to aid in minimizing connective tissue injury.

## REFERENCES

1. Adams, Adran. "Effect of Exercise on Ligament Strength." *Research Quarterly* 37 (1966) :163.

2. Adams, R. D.; Brown, Denny; and Pearson, C. M. *Diseases of Muscle.* New York: Paul B. Hoeber, 1962.

3. Billig, H. E. *Mobilization of the Human Body.* Palo Alto, Calif.: Stanford University Press, 1941.

4. Broer, Marion R. *An Introduction to Kinesiology.* Englewood Cliffs, N.J.: Prentice-Hall, 1968.

5. Committee on Medical Rating of Physical Impairment. "Guide to the Evaluation of Permanent Impairment of the Back and Extremities." *Journal of the American Medical Association* 16 (1958) :1.

6. deVries, H. A. "Evaluation of Static Stretching Procedures for Improvement of Flexibility." *Research Quarterly* 33 (1962) :222.

7. Gardner, E. "Physiology of Moveable Joints." *Physiology Review 30 (1959):127.*

8. Holland, George J. "The Physiology of Flexibility, A Review of the Literature." *Kinesiology Review* 1 (1968) :49.

9. Kottke, F. J., and Mundale, M. A. "Range of Mobility of the Cervical Spine." *Archives of Physical Medicine* 40 (1959) :379.

10. Kraus, H., and Raab, W. *Hypokinetic Disease, Diseases Produced by Lack of Exercise.* Springfield, Ill.: Charles C Thomas, 1961.

11. Leighton, J. R. "On the Significance of Flexibility for Physical Education." *Journal of Health, Physical Education, Recreation* 31 (1960) :27.

12. Parry, C. B. "Stretching." In *Massage, Manipulation and Traction,* edited by S. Licht. New Haven: Elizabeth Licht, Publisher, 1960.

13. Vernado, A., and LaCava, G. "Footballer's Ankle." *Lancet* 2 (1964) :694.

# 10 | Biologic Bases of Cardiorespiratory Endurance

THE FIRST two chapters of Part 4 have been concerned with the biological bases of flexibility and muscular strength. It should be remembered that strength training is concerned with improving man's performance of short-term muscular events. The present chapter is concerned with the major physiological systems involved in supporting man's performance of sustained muscular work. Conceivably it is possible for an individual to possess very large (hypertrophied) and very strong muscles for performing muscular feats requiring only several seconds of muscular contraction and yet have very little physiological reserve for the performance of endurance activities. Such an individual would lack the necessary adaptations in his cardiovascular and respiratory systems to sustain prolonged work, such as that required for distance running, bicycling or swimming, or participation in vigorous recreational activities such as tennis, badminton, basketball, handball, soccer and the like. Insofar as directness of relationship to one's organic vigor and physical health is concerned, however, cardiorespiratory endurance is of much greater significance than any other dimension of fitness.

## DEFINITION OF ENDURANCE

Cardiorespiratory endurance is the ability to efficiently use the large body muscles in repetitive or sustained muscular contractions for relatively long periods of time. From a physiological point of view, cardiorespiratory efficiency implies the ability to participate in endurance activities without undue fatigue and to recover quickly upon the cessation of exercise. The ability to conduct endurance work without excessive fatigue and with rapid recovery is the result of biological adaptation within many of the physiological systems. Essentially, however, all endurance work is dependent upon the delivery of an increased $O_2$ supply to the working muscle cells in order to support the greatly increased metabolization of carbohydrates (glucose). As pointed out in Chapter 7, man has only a very limited capacity to work anaerobically and develop oxygen debt, i.e., metabolize glucose without $O_2$. We may think practically, therefore, of man's oxygen transport capacity (maximum oxygen consumption) as being synonomous with his endurance work capacity. Efficient oxygen transport capacity during exercise and the subsequent recovery period is primarily dependent upon the functions of the lungs, heart, and blood vessels.

### PULMONARY FUNCTION

The pulmonary system transfers the atmospheric $O_2$ to the pulmonary blood through the function known as external respiration. To accomplish this, large volumes of air must be moved through the pulmonary system each minute since the atmosphere contains only about 20 percent $O_2$, and only a fraction of that diffuses into the blood with each inhalation. At rest approximately 6.0 liters of air are moved in and out of the lungs each minute. This measure is designated as pulmonary ventilation and is primarily dependent upon the work of the diaphragm and intercostal muscles. During exercise the pulmonary ventilation may increase in well-trained athletes to as much as 200 liters/minute (24). With the high pulmonary ventilation during heavy exercise, the energy cost per liter ventilation becomes progressively greater, and the oxygen cost of breathing may be up to 10 percent of the body's total working oxygen requirement (18).

Man's ability to achieve very high levels of oxygen consumption to support high level endurance work is highly correlated with his pulmonary ventilatory capacity. In this respect, it should be noted that normal cigarette smoking causes (within several seconds) a several-fold increase in the airway resistance of the pulmonary system (6). This narrowing effect of nicotine and tobacco particles upon the airway passages will necessarily create increased impedance to air flow and normal pulmonary ventilation during endurance exercise. Holland and Rich (12) have provided a comprehensive review of the effects of smoking on physiological work efficiency.

Laboratory techniques have been developed to determine the rate at which $O_2$ and $CO_2$ diffuse between the alveolar air of the lungs and the pulmonary capillary blood of the lungs. The rate of diffusion of these gases through the tissue membranes is, of course, dependent upon the differential partial pressure of the two gases. According to Astrand, pulmonary diffusion rate is also dependent upon the total alveolar surface area (which is related to total lung size), absence of fibrosis or thickening of the tissue membrane separating alveolar air from pulmonary blood, as with the condition of emphysema, and the total pulmonary blood volume (2). The pulmonary blood volume increases significantly during exercise due to the number of open or dilated capillaries and is primarily responsible for increases above the resting pulmonary diffusion rate in trained endurance athletes of as much as 200 percent (13). With increasing age in adults, the pulmonary diffusing capacity is significantly reduced (10).

### CARDIOVASCULAR FUNCTION

Once $O_2$ has diffused from the alveoli to the pulmonary blood and attached itself to the hemoglobin of the red blood cells, it must be transported to the working muscle cells to support sustained muscular contractions during endurance activity. This transport function is accomplished by the heart and blood vessels. Certain metabolic byproducts, such as $CO_2$ and heat, are transported by the cardiovascular system from the working muscle cells to other anatomical sites (the lungs, for example) where they can be dissipated or removed from the body.

The most important modification in cardiovascular function during endurance exercise is that of cardiac output, i.e., the total volume of blood expelled by one side of the heart each minute. This may be accomplished by increasing the number of heart beats per minute and/or increasing the amount of blood pumped out of the heart (stroke volume) during each contraction or systole. Generally, the heart rate increases during maximum exercise up to about two and one half times the resting value; rarely, however, in normal subjects does it exceed 200 beats per minute (5). There is a gradual decline in maximal heart rate with age, the sixty-five-year-old attaining only about 165 beats per minute (21). How rapidly the heart rate returns to approximately the preexercise or resting level is one important index of cardiovascular efficiency. Stroke volume also increases significantly during prolonged exercise, usually anywhere from 30 percent to 50 percent (3). These increases in stroke volume are due primarily to increased power of contraction by the heart muscle (3, 23). This kind of sustained work by the heart during endurance exercise has many implications for cardiovascular health. These biological implications account for the strong emphasis on cardiorespiratory endurance activities in modern physical fitness programs.

If man engages in vigorous muscular activity for several minutes or longer, profound changes in blood flow to the various tissues occur. This is due to the drastically increased demand for $O_2$ (and, therefore, blood) in some tissues such as muscle, and a decreased priority for blood flow in other inactive tissue such as the viscera. Under specific exercise conditions, certain muscles may gain almost a 50 percent increase in blood flow (15). This is, of course, necessary to support the high rate of energy metabolism in muscles engaged in endurance work. These dramatic shifts in blood flow during exercise are accomplished by selective vasoconstriction (narrowing) and vasodilation (relaxation) of the arterial blood vessels. There is pervasive arterial vasodilation in the skeletal muscles of man during prolonged endurance exercise along with vasoconstriction in the inactive tissues of the body such as the brain, skeleton and viscera. In addition, valves at the head of the muscle capillaries (precapillary sphincters) open up following stimulus by exercise metabolites such as $CO_2$ to permit greater blood perfusion of the muscle tissue.

The adaptive vasoconstrictive and vasodilative ability of the arteries is due to the presence of smooth muscle in the middle layer of these vessels. This arterial smooth muscle is under autonomic nervous system control and plays a very important role in the differential shunting of blood during endurance activities. It is assumed that the stress we impose on our blood vessels during regular exercise (as evidenced by changes in blood pressure) is important to their biological integrity. In very practical terms we can think of endurance activities as providing an exercise stress not only for our skeletal muscles, but also for the smooth muscles of our arterial blood vessels. Rohter et al. (22) have reported significant increases in exercise blood flow through the forearm muscles after six weeks of endurance swimming training.

## IMPORTANCE OF CARDIORESPIRATORY ENDURANCE

Attention has already been directed to certain physiological rationale regarding the importance of cardiorespiratory endurance to one's overall physical health. Essentially, endurance activities provide a significant stimulus to the heart muscle (myocardium) and the smooth muscle of the blood vessels, as well as the entire pulmonary system.

Boyer has summarized the major physiological changes associated with long-term training: lower resting and working heart rate, an increase in resting and working heart rate, an increase in resting and exercise stroke volume, an increase in maximum cardiac output, an increase in velocity of myocardial contraction, increase in size (hypertrophy) of the heart muscle, a decrease in systemic arterial blood pressure, and a redistribution of blood flow to the more active muscles (4). Thus, regular conditioning in endurance activities provides the individual with a "physiological reserve" to face any emergency of prolonged duration.

Endurance trained individuals have lower resting, exercise and recovery heart rates and blood pressure, along with increased pulmonary capacity. Such individuals show higher working capacity (aerobic capacity) when measured under standard laboratory conditions and thus open avenues of recreational pursuit which are quite unlimited. With a lower propensity for physical fatigue, they can presumably conduct a normal day's work with little undue stress upon their physiological systems. Most importantly, they possess a reserve capacity which permits them maximum vitality and enjoyment in any physical dimension. In addition, endurance activities require significant levels of caloric expenditure and thus may be used as part of a weight reduction or weight control program.

## PLANNING ENDURANCE CONDITIONING ACTIVITIES

The types of physical activities which provide sufficient physiological stimulus for improvement of cardiorespiratory endurance are quite varied. In Figures 10.1 and 10.2, laboratory methods are illustrated using the running treadmill and bicycle ergometer for measuring maximum work capacity. The subject runs or pedals until he or she reaches maximum or near maximum (submaximum) heart rate and oxygen consumption. When training in the laboratory to improve one's performance on these endurance tests, the work rate and duration on the treadmill or bicycle are gradually increased over a period of many weeks. In this way the individual becomes accustomed and adjusted to the gradually increased stress and discomfort which is imposed upon his physiology. Much more informal approaches can be utilized outside the laboratory in a wide variety of endurance activities, providing that certain basic training principles are adhered to.

Running, cycling or swimming probably represents the ideal method for regular endurance training because these activities do not require extensive training facilities and can be accomplished in a minimum of time. Such activities are ideal for the person initiating a conditioning program or attempting to recondition himself after a considerable period of seden-

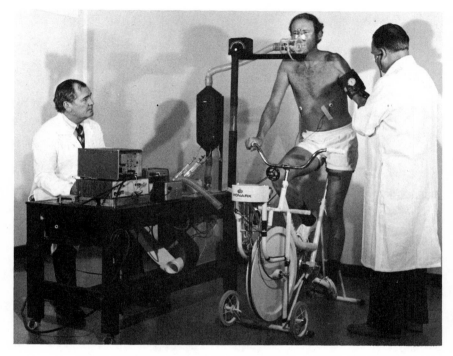

*FIGURE 10.1    Endurance Testing, Bicycle Ergometer*

tary living, since the total amount of work can be estimated at each training session. This allows the individual to carefully plan a graded intensity
program which is both safe and effective in achieving his desired goals
of endurance fitness.

After achieving a good physiological "endurance base," which usually
requires several months in the case of a poorly conditioned person, a
wider variety of endurance activities which are of interest to and provide
recreational enjoyment and competition for the participant may be followed. Participation in any endurance training activities should be pursued
only after medical assessment of one's physiological tolerance for such
activity and must follow safe and sound principles of training. General
principles of endurance conditioning are considered below and should be
carefully studied by the individual planning such a program.

*Medical Clearance.*    Probably no other conditioning activities stress
the total physiology as dramatically as those designed to improve endurance. Because of this, no adult should begin an endurance training pro-

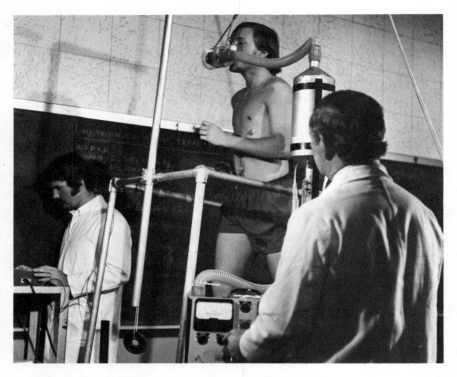

*FIGURE 10.2    Endurance Testing, Treadmill Ergometer*

gram without first consulting a physician and undergoing a comprehensive medical screening. Such screening should give particular emphasis to pulmonary and cardiovascular function. It is the consensus of leading cardiologists that an exercise stress electrocardiogram should be included in the examination (*19, 25*). Clinical examination of the exercise stress electrocardiogram often uncovers functional heart disease that may preclude one's participation in vigorous physical activity. It is particularly important for the person who has been sedentary for many years to seek such medical screening and consult with the physician regarding his planned program of activities.

   *Progression.*    A carefully planned program of increasing intensity should be outlined prior to initiation of the training sessions. The beginning level of training will be dependent upon prior conditioning and general state of health. The individual who has been very sedentary for several years may wish to begin with only light stretching calisthenic activities for several minutes each day, designed to only slightly increase the breathing and heart rate (see Chap. 9). As one becomes accustomed to this level of work, he or she may begin walking in place or outdoors for specified periods of time, gradually increasing the distance and pace (rate and duration of work). Eventually, the endurance work stress shall consist of jogging in place or over a course of set distance. If running outdoors hard surfaces such as asphalt and concrete should be avoided in favor of a turf or grass surface. Also, good running shoes with a thick soft sole should be used to absorb shock and minimize leg injuries. If confined to indoors, many persons effectively increase the work load by stepping up and down on a solidly based chair or stool. It should be recognized that such activity is quite strenuous and should not be engaged in as a beginning conditioning activity. Metabolically, it is comparable to running at a moderate pace.

Only after many weeks of low intensity work would the conditioning activities be increased to the level where the individual is conscious of even moderate physiological discomfort. In addition to the discomfort which one feels during and after endurance exercise, the amount of time spent exercising and the work rate can be utilized in assessing one's graded progression. An important point to remember is that it is always better to progress too slowly, rather than too fast, in an endurance fitness program. This is particularly important with increasing age. In fact, the middle-aged or older person should spend many weeks in very low-level calisthenic and walking activities before jogging or participating in similar activities for even short periods of time.

In this discussion of the principle of endurance progression, primary emphasis has been given to walking and the eventual goals of jogging and running. The same guidelines discussed in this respect could be applied to bicycling or endurance swimming, careful attention being given to work rate and duration. Stationary bicycles are available which may be conveniently used in the home or office and permit easy assessment of rate as well as work intensity. Such bicycle ergometers are a convenient and relatively inexpensive facility for endurance conditioning which can be used the year round.

*Optimum Training Stimulus.* The number of training sessions per week in order to significantly improve endurance function is somewhat controvertible. Massie and Shephard (16) demonstrated in sedentary middle-aged men that predicted aerobic power (maximum oxygen consumption during exercise) increased 10 percent in twenty-eight weeks with three 20-minute sessions of vigorous exercise per week. Total body weight and percent of body fat can be significantly reduced by a three-day, ten-week program of moderate jogging (26). Significant improvement in most indices of physical fitness can be expected in a fifteen-week program of conditioning for young, healthy college students (9). Training sessions may be limited to two per week, but more optimum results can be expected with three (8). Kasch and Carter (14) reported that physiological manifestations of endurance training effects show a leveling effect after approximately one year of training.

Each individual must ascertain within the limits of available time and motivation how much time he can devote to his or her endurance conditioning program. As one progressively increases the intensity of the work stimulu⁻, it becomes necessary to work for short periods of time and intersperse such work periods with rest. This approach makes use of the interval training concept and permits the individual to prolong the overall training session without undue fatigue. Cooper (7) has estimated that for optimum endurance training effect a heart rate of at least 150 must be sustained for five minutes or longer. Kasch and Carter (14) recommend that at least 70 percent of the maximum working heart rate be utilized as the optimum training stimulus for middle-aged males. Many months may be required before very sedentary individuals can achieve a working heart rate of that magnitude. Hellerstein (11) recommends much lower working heart rates with increasing age, never exceeding 85 percent of the predicted maximum.

At no time is it recommended that "all out" endurance activity, approaching maximum heart rates, be utilized in the layman's endurance fitness training program. Excessive levels of physiological discomfort are not necessary to provide sufficient stimulus for improvement of physiological endurance. This is one reason why poorly conditioned persons should avoid competitive endurance training for the first several months. It eventually becomes necessary for the sedentary person planning his own endurance conditioning program to learn to use his own exercise heart rate as an index of physiological stress and training.

It is practically impossible to palpitate one's heart rate while exercising, but quite simple while at rest. The pulse at the neck (carotid) or wrist (radial) may be utilized. In assessing exercise heart rate it is important to obtain it as soon as possible after the cessation of exercise. Fifteen-second heart rate later multiplied by four will provide a quick index of the work load imposed on the total physiology. By charting several minutes of pre-exercise resting heart rate, immediate postexercise heart rate and recovery heart rate (until it returns to approximately the preexercise level), a fairly reliable index of the physiological endurance efficiency may be achieved. Periodically, such evaluation of cardiovascular work efficiency should be conducted under conditions as standard as possible. Standard step tests, which impose a constant work load on your muscles and physiological systems, have been developed (see Figure 10.3). Usually, benches of 18 inches for men and 16 inches for women are recommended. Benches of 12 inches are recommended for middle-aged and older persons (20). Normative data on heart rate recovery for different age groups may be referred to (17). Any similar short-term work stress test may be used to assess physiological efficiency through recovery heart rate. Persons who train for many months in endurance activities usually show significant decrease in resting, postexercise, and recovery heart rates.

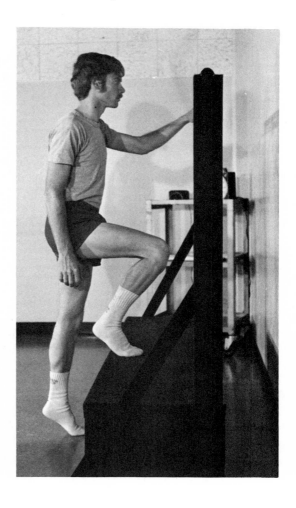

FIGURE 10.3   Cardiovas-
cular Step Test

*Warm-Up.*   Before participating in endurance activities for fitness purposes there are several reasons for warming up. Warming up may consist of stretching, followed by very light walking and jogging, or very light bouts of pedaling on the bicycle, before any strenuous exertion. Essentially, such warm-up slightly raises body temperature and allows the metabolic processes in the cell to proceed at a higher rate, since such processes are temperature-dependent. With increased body temperature, oxygenation of the muscle cells is also enhanced. Physical work capacity is also increased following warm-up (1). Maximum benefits are experienced after fifteen minutes of warm-up, although five minutes of low-level warm-up is sufficient for participation in ordinary endurance activities (2). With limited data, deVries (8) has presented perhaps one of the most practical reasons for warm-up, and that is prevention of connective tissue injury. It is this author's opinion, based upon experience with various adult fitness programs, that with increasing age the period of warm-up must be proportionately increased in order to minimize the possibility of muscle and other connective tissue injuries.

Following completion of an endurance training session it is further recommended that gradual "cooling down" be followed. This is a kind of reverse warm-up in which the individual gradually tapers off his energy expenditure until after five or ten minutes he begins to approach the pre-exercise or resting level. Cooling down, and warm-up, help the person pursuing an endurance conditioning program avoid acute and dramatic shifts in the physiological stress imposed upon the body systems. Such procedures allow the pulmonary, cardiovascular and metabolic processes to slowly return to the resting or basal level.

## SUMMARY

Endurance training is directed towards improvement of the functional efficiency of the physiological systems which support man's sustained muscular work. Endurance work performance is primarily dependent upon the coordinated function of the pulmonary and cardiovascular systems to support the skeletal muscle cell metabolism. Long-term endurance training results in larger maximum oxygen consumption, pulmonary ventilation, and pulmonary diffusion. The endurance trained individual also has a higher cardiac blood volume output (cardiac output), and because of this demonstrates lower resting, working and recovery heart rates and blood pressures than sedentary persons. The quantitative changes in cardiovascular function which occur as a result of endurance conditioning undoubtedly could play a significant role in the prevention of coronary heart disease. Endurance reconditioning programs should be carefully developed with safe gradation of stress imposed upon the sedentary person's physiological systems.

The biological outcomes described in the last three chapters, because of their benefit to man, become personal values to her or him who is willing to pay the price. The values of physical activity to man throughout history have ranged from survival (early man) to pure recreation (modern man). Today, man's radically altered physical life-style is controverting his innate biological demand for physical activity. Planning for the biological outcomes of physical activity requires weaving these values into one's personal system of values. Guidelines have been presented for the development of balanced longitudinal programs which emphasize desirable biological outcomes.

## REFERENCES

1. Asmussen, E., and Boje, O. "Body Temperature and Capacity for Work." *Acta Physiol. Scand.* 10 (1945):1.

2. Astrand, P. O. and Rodahl, K. *Textbook of Work Physiology.* New York: McGraw-Hill, 1970, p. 222.

3. Astrand, P. O.; Cuddy, T. E.; Saltin, B.; and Steinberg, J. "Cardiac Output During Submaximal and Maximal Work." *Journal of Applied Physiology* 19 (1964):268.

4. Boyer, John M. "Effects of Chronic Exercise on Cardiovascular Function." In *Physical Fitness Research Digest.* President's Council on Physical Fitness and Sports, ser. 2, no. 3, July 1972.

5. Brouha, L., and Radford, E. P. "The Cardiovascular System in Muscular Activity." In *Science and Medicine of Sports,* edited by W. R. Johnson. New York: Harper & Brothers, 1960, p. 187.

6. Comroe, J. H. "The Lung." *Scientific American* 214 (1966):56.

7. Cooper, K. H. *Aerobics.* New York: Evans Publ. Co., 1968.

8. deVries, H. A. *Physiology of Exercise.* Dubuque, Iowa: Wm. C. Brown Co., 1974.

9. deVries, H. A., and Bartlett, K. T. "Effects of a Minimal Time Conditioning Program Upon Selected Motor Fitness Measures of College Men." *Journal of the Association for Physical and Mental Rehabilitation* 16 (1962):99–102.

10. Donevan, R. E.; Palmer, W. H.; Varvis, C. J.; and Bates, D. V. "Influence of Age on Pulmonary Diffusing Capacity." *Journal of Applied Physiology* 14 (1959):483.

11. Hellerstein, H. K. "Exercise and the Treatment of Heart Disease." *Journal of the South Carolina Medical Association* 65 (December 1969):46–56.

12. Holland, George, and Rich, III, G. Q. "Implications for Human Performance from Research Studies on the Physiology of Smoking." *Oregon Association for Health, Physical Education and Recreation Journal* 3 (February 1969):10.

13. Holmgren, A., and Astrand, P. O. "D.L. and the Dimensions and Functional Ca-

pacities of the $O_2$ Transport System on Humans." *Journal of Applied Physiology* 21 (1966):1463.

14. Kasch, F. W., and Carter, J. E. L. "Training Patterns in Middle-Aged Males." *Journal of Sports Medicine and Physical Fitness* 10 (December 1970):225.

15. Martin, E. G.; Wooley, E. C.; and Miller, M. "Capillary Counts in Resting and Active Muscle." *American Journal of Physiology* 100 (1932):407–16.

16. Massie, J. F., and Shephard, R. J. "Physical and Physiological Effects of Training." *Medicine and Science in Sports* 3 (1971):110–17.

17. Michael, E. M., and Gallon, A. "Periodic Changes in the Circulation During Athletic Training as Reflected by a Step Test." *Research Quarterly* 30 (1959):303–11.

18. Otis, A. B., "The Work of Breathing," in *Handbook of Physiology*, edited by W. O. Finn and H. Rohns. Washington: American Physiological Society, 1964.

19. Parmley, L. F., ed. "Proceedings of the National Workshop on Exercise in the Prevention, in the Evaluation, in the Treatment of Heart Disease." *Journal of South Carolina Medical Association* 65 (December 1969):1.

20. Preventive Medicine Institute. *Health Enhancement Through Physical Activity.* Palo Alto, Calif.: Preventive Medicine Institute, 1970.

21. Robinson, S. "Experimental Studies of Physical Fitness in Relation to Age." *Arbeitsphysiol* 10 (1938):251.

22. Rohter, F. D.; Rochelle, R. H.; and Hyman, C. "Exercise Blood Flow Changes in the Human Forearm During Physical Training." *Journal of Applied Physiology* 18 (1963):789–93.

23. Rushmer, R. F. "Regulation of the Heart's Function." *Circulation* 21 (1960):744.

24. Saltin, B., and Astrand, P. O. "Maximal Oxygen Uptake in Athletes." *Journal of Applied Physiology* 23 (1967):353.

25. Shephard, R. J., Chm. and ed. "Proceedings of the International Symposium on Physical Activity and Cardiovascular Health." *Journal of the Canadian Medical Association* 96 (March 1967):695.

26. Wilmore, J.; Royce, J.; Guandola, R.; Katch, F.; and Katch, V. "Body Composition Changes with a Ten-Week Program of Jogging." *Medicine and Science in Sports* 3 (1970): 113–17.

# Index